CONDUCTING RESEARCH IN THE PRACTICE SETTING

RESEARCH METHODS FOR PRIMARY CARE

The goal of RESEARCH METHODS FOR PRIMARY CARE is to address important topics meeting the needs of the growing number of primary care researchers. Purposely following a sequence from general principles to specific techniques, implementation strategies, and dissemination, the series volumes each examine a particular aspect of primary care research, emphasizing actually conducting research in the real world. The well-known contributors bring an international, multidisciplinary perspective to the volumes, enhancing their usefulness to primary care researchers.

Volumes in the series:

1. **Primary Care Research: Traditional and Innovative Approaches**
   Edited by Peter G. Norton, Moira Stewart, Fred Tudiver, Martin J. Bass, and Earl V. Dunn

2. **Tools for Primary Care Research**
   Edited by Moira Stewart, Fred Tudiver, Martin J. Bass, Earl V. Dunn, and Peter G. Norton

3. **Doing Qualitative Research**
   Edited by Benjamin F. Crabtree and William L. Miller

4. **Assessing Interventions: Traditional and Innovative Methods**
   Edited by Fred Tudiver, Martin J. Bass, Earl V. Dunn, Peter G. Norton, and Moira Stewart

5. **Conducting Research in the Practice Setting**
   Edited by Martin J. Bass, Earl V. Dunn, Peter G. Norton, Moira Stewart, and Fred Tudiver

Forthcoming title in the series includes:

6. **Disseminating New Knowledge and Having an Impact on Practice**
   Edited by Earl V. Dunn, Peter G. Norton, Moira Stewart, Fred Tudiver, and Martin J. Bass

CONDUCTING RESEARCH IN THE PRACTICE SETTING

EDITED BY

MARTIN J. BASS
EARL V. DUNN
PETER G. NORTON
MOIRA STEWART
FRED TUDIVER

Research Methods
for Primary Care
Volume 5

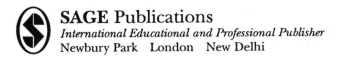

SAGE Publications
International Educational and Professional Publisher
Newbury Park   London   New Delhi

Copyright © 1993 by Sage Publications, Inc.

For information address:

SAGE Publications, Inc.
2455 Teller Road
Newbury Park, California 91320

SAGE Publications Ltd.
6 Bonhill Street
London EC2A 4PU
United Kingdom

SAGE Publications India Pvt. Ltd.
M-32 Market
Greater Kailash I
New Delhi 110 048 India

Printed in the United States of America

Library of Congress Cataloging-in-Publication Data

Main entry under title:

Conducting research in the practice setting / edited by Martin J. Bass
 . . . [et al.].
        p.   cm.   — (Research methods for primary care; v. 5)
    Includes bibliographical references and index.
    ISBN 0-8039-5126-4 (cl.)   — ISBN 0-8039-5127-2 (pb)
    1. Primary health care—Research—Methodology. I. Bass, Martin
J. II. Series.
    [DNLM: 1. Research—methods. 2. Primary Health Care. 3. Family
Practice.   W1 RE232C v.5 1993]
    R850.C656   1993
    610'.72—dc20
    DNLM/DLC   93-973

93 94 95 96   10 9 8 7 6 5 4 3 2 1

Sage Production Editor: Diane S. Foster

Contents

112102

Foreword: Conducting Research in the Practice Setting

PAUL A. NUTTING

The products of the last decade of health services research have shown us how little we really know about what we do in medical care that actually benefits our patients. Although there are many individual findings, the most dramatic point to the unexplained variations that exist in services used across small geographic areas. As early as 1938, John Glover (1938), in England, reported a 10-fold difference in rates of tonsillectomy among different areas. Since then, several developed countries—notably Canada, the United States, and England—have documented dramatic variation in hospital admission, lengths of hospital stay, and specific surgical procedures (Bunker, 1970; Chassin et al., 1986; Roos & Roos, 1981; Stockwell & Vayda, 1979; Vayda, 1973; Wennberg, 1984; Wennberg & Gittlesohn, 1973). The presence of practice variation is assumed to reflect ambiguity about the effectiveness of major components of medical care and has spawned a major research initiative and a new agency of the U.S. Public Health Service to coordinate that research (Agency for Health Care Policy and Research, 1990).

However long overdue, one wonders why now, in the 1990s, we need a new major research initiative to understand the effectiveness of all we have learned after a half-century of heavy investment in medical research. In my view, this situation points to the important limitations of the biomedical research model that has driven research since the late 1940s. This model has produced incredible knowledge about the mechanisms of disease and the processes that mediate treatment, but it has produced less to guide us in the practice of medicine and especially the primary care of our patients.

More than 30 years ago, Kerr White described the ecology of medical care and changed the way we think about the linkage between primary care and the health care needs of the population (White, Williams, & Greenberg, 1961). Applying data from national surveys to a hypothetical population of 1,000 adults in the community, he showed that approximately three-quarters, or 750 individuals, would report one or more illnesses during a given month. Of these, approximately one-third, or 250 people, would seek care from their physician. Nine would be admitted to a community hospital, five would be referred to another physician, and only one would be admitted to a tertiary care hospital. This example puts into perspective the relative magnitudes of the population's need for health services and has been confirmed by more contemporary estimates (Thacker, Greene, & Salber, 1977). Roughly 25% of the population seeks physician care in a given month, yet only 0.9% require hospitalization or specialty care, and only 0.1% require tertiary care services.

Although less than 1% of the population receives care in the specialty sector, it is in this setting that the majority of research is done. This setting is appropriate for research that expands the frontiers of our understanding of the basic mechanisms of disease and of those that mediate treatment. However, this alone is not adequate to inform decisions that must be made for the patients and their problems that present to the family physician. The powerful selection bias that results from both medical and self-referral concentrates patients in subspecialty centers with diseases very different from the undifferentiated illnesses seen in primary care (McWhinney, 1981).

Most current biomedical research carefully restricts the range of issues under study in several important ways. First, most studies isolate single diseases or disease processes in order to study specific disease in its fully developed form in patients, without other conditions that would confound the study. In many cases a specific organ, tissue, cell, or intracellular process is the focus of study. Second, disease is studied in highly selected patients. To focus on a specific disease mechanism or treatment effect, most medical research carefully restricts the characteristics of the patients under study to persons in their middle years, without other comorbidity, and in whom compliance can be carefully controlled. Third, most medical research is designed to evaluate single interventions. Although many clinical trials compare several interventions, they rarely are combined in a single arm of the trial in ways they are actually used in our practices. Fourth, most studies use "hard" outcomes, such as death and change in measurable physical parameters. Relatively little attention is devoted to key personal consequences of effective primary care, such as relief of suffering, a sense of having been understood, vitality, the preservation and restoration of function, and the quality of well-being. Finally, most clinical trials systematically exclude the effects of the patients' physical and psychosocial environments, the powerful effects of the patient-physician relationship, and the multiple effects of the system factors inherent in the organization and financing of health care services.

Nonetheless the value of traditional biomedical research is unquestioned. It has led to critically important advances in diagnostic and treatment technologies. It has not, however, translated well into practice to support the decisions that family physicians must make in the care of patients who suffer from undifferentiated illnesses, embedded in the psychosocial context of their lives. Additional research is needed that focuses on the patients and problems of primary care and that accommodates the variety of settings that typify primary care in North America. It is in practice settings that much of the important work can be accomplished to complete our understanding of the clinical spectrum of illness as it affects most people in the community most of the time.

Our success in basic biomedical research is due in no small part to more than 200 major, tertiary care hospitals in the United States and Canada, where specialty care, teaching, and research are conducted. These institutions provide the infrastructure for our biomedical research enterprise, structured to provide access to patients and their disease and the technology necessary to describe the diseases that are the focus of the research mission of the institutions. To study the relevant phenomena of primary care, however, is a logistical problem. There are no comparable institutions in the unselected populations and problems that present to the primary care physician.

To observe the relevant phenomena of family practice and primary care, we must develop laboratories outside the tertiary care centers. Practice-based research networks have emerged over the last decade for just this purpose. These organizations link practicing primary care physicians with the research expertise required to design and conduct research on the diagnosis and management of the common problems people bring to their family physician. They also provide the rudiments of an infrastructure and provide access to the relevant phenomena of primary care.

Despite our enthusiasm, a great deal remains yet to be done. We are poised at the beginning of a new era in health care research and face important challenges in framing the relevant research questions and in developing and adapting methods that will produce information useful in practice. Martin Bass and his colleagues have assembled another volume in this remarkable series to deal with the practical issues in conducting research in practice settings. The volume recognizes that research in primary care must be driven, not by our favorite methods, but by the relevant questions that emerge from the care of our patients. Thus research in family practice and primary care requires effective collaboration across several settings, disciplines, and institutional bases. Similarly the chapter authors stress the critical importance of qualitative research and the role of qualitative methods in matching the research question to the research approach. Recognizing that primary care settings will vary as widely as the populations they serve, this volume describes research opportunities in practice settings that range widely, including Native American, homeless, rural, as well as suburban communities. In compiling Volume 5 in the series, Bass and his colleagues have shown us the direction and have provided strategies for systematic inquiry into the important elements of our work. The information contained herein will prove invaluable to all researchers striving to advance the scientific underpinnings of primary care practice.

References

Agency for Health Care Policy and Research. (1990). *Medical treatment effectiveness research* (Agency for Health Care Policy and Research Program Note). Rockville, MD: Department of Health and Human Services, Public Health Service.

Bunker, J. P. (1970). Surgical manpower: A comparison of operations and surgeons in the United States and in England and Wales. *New England Journal of Medicine, 282,* 135-144.

Chassin, M. R., Brook, R. H., Park, R. E., Keesey, J., Fink, A., Kosecoff, J., Kahn, K., Merrick, N., & Solomon, D. H. (1986). Variations in the use of medical and surgical services by the Medicare population. *New England Journal of Medicine, 314,* 285-290.

Glover, J. A. (1938). The incidence of tonsillectomy in school children. *Proceedings of the Royal Society of Medicine, 31,* 1219-1236.

McWhinney, I. R. (1981). *An introduction to family medicine.* New York: Oxford University Press.

Roos, N. P., & Roos, L. L. (1981). High and low surgical rates: Risk factors for area residents. *American Journal of Public Health, 71,* 591-600.

Stockwell, J., & Vayda, E. (1979). Variations in surgery in Ontario. *Medical Care, 17,* 390-396.

Thacker, S. B., Greene, S. B., & Salber, E. J. (1977). Hospitalizations in a Southern rural community: An application of the "ecology model." *International Journal of Epidemiology, 6,* 55-63.

Vayda, E. (1973). A comparison of surgical rates in Canada and in England and Wales. *New England Journal of Medicine, 289,* 1224-1229.

Wennberg, J. (1984). Dealing with medical practice variations: A proposal for action. *Health Affairs, 3,* 6-32.

Wennberg, J., & Gittlesohn, A. (1973). Small area variations in health care delivery. *Science, 182,* 1102-1108.

White, K. L., Williams, T. F., & Greenberg, B. G. (1961). The ecology of medical care. *New England Journal of Medicine, 265,* 885-892.

Acknowledgments

The editors thank the Physicians' Services Incorporated Foundation, Ontario, for their generous support for the production of this volume. They also thank the National Health Research and Development Program (NHRDP) of the Federal Government of Canada for financial support. Anne Stilman's able editing improved the manuscript markedly. The tireless efforts of Vanessa Orr and Sandra Richard-Mohamed enabled this book to become a reality.

Introduction

MARTIN J. BASS

The practice setting is the laboratory of primary care research. This is where the primary care provider and the patient interact, whether it be in the provider's office, the patient's home, or one of the less frequent sites such as the nursing home, the school, or even the street. Because the models of in-hospital and traditional laboratory research are not useful for primary care, new approaches with new variables and outcomes are essential. In this volume we have assembled the reflections and studies of 24 experienced primary care researchers from the fields of family practice and nursing. Through sharing examples of their work, they have identified the methods and elements necessary for conducting successful primary care research.

As in the previous volumes of this series, the authors are international (Canada, United States, United Kingdom, and Israel) and multidisciplinary (family medicine, nursing, social work, epidemiology, and anthropology). The research approaches discussed include both quantitative and qualitative methods as they apply to the primary care setting.

The book is divided into four parts. Part I considers general issues of primary care research. One chapter provides an innovative framework for organizing the many types of primary care research. Another chapter addresses the important issue of quality research by identifying predisposing, enabling, and reinforcing factors. A third considers the always-present ethical issues when conducting research with human subjects, which are even more complex when those subjects have an ongoing relationship with the researcher as patients. All three chapters in this section introduce themes that recur throughout the book: the importance of collaboration, the necessity for qualitative and quantitative methods, and the practical nature of primary care research.

Part II primarily deals with the practical issues of conducting research in the office setting. These issues include combining clinical care and research, recruiting patients, using qualitative approaches, making maximum use of the office computer, and identifying the needs of the surrounding community.

Part III expands on the theme of collaboration, with chapters on nurse/physician collaboration, physician within networks, industry/provider collaboration, and university/community collaboration.

Part IV deals with special settings for primary care research. A variety of settings that are relevant to primary care present distinct research challenges. Because of page limitations, we were able to focus on only five settings. We hope that those chosen will draw attention to overlooked areas and will present new challenges and ideas to the reader. The chapters in Part IV cover rural native communities, the homeless, the teaching setting, long-term care settings, and the community.

The final section of the book, an appendix, is a checklist for conducting research in the practice setting. We appreciate that readers will have a range of experience in research from beginner to accomplished. For those readers wanting to know how to conduct research in their practice setting and who consequently were drawn to this volume by its title, this checklist will be a useful framework and guide. To be of value, primary care research must meet the standards that are summarized in the checklist.

We hope this book will assist and encourage primary care practitioners in conducting research in their practice setting.

PART I

General Issues

1 A Research Strategy for Family Medicine: Pure or Applied?

NIGEL C. H. STOTT

> The scientific process has two motives: one to understand the natural world, the other to control it.
>
> C. P. Snow (1964, p. 10)

International strategic thinking on health services has had a 25-year gestation but is now firmly on the agenda of most nation-states. The World Health Organization's (1978) call for "Health for All by the Year 2000" has been converted into wide-ranging health targets, and many countries are involved in producing local health strategies in an attempt to meet these targets. The major themes that have emerged from these strategic exercises are as follows:

1. To redress some of the huge differences in life and health expectancy between and within countries
2. To shift the emphasis in health care toward more health promotion
3. To identify governmental responsibility for healthful environments (e.g., water, air, food, housing)
4. To build formal health services on a foundation of primary health care, targeting resources to areas of most need
5. To develop a "research culture" in every health service

The success of these initiatives is regarded as needing not only central direction in each country but also involvement of

3

a wide range of agencies, including "the people" in their own communities. This "top-down/bottom-up" approach is likely to cause maximum stress at the interfaces between the public and the formal health service: the primary care interface. Here traditional attitudes and beliefs will meet the new health culture at a personal level, and both the public and the professional staff are being exhorted to trade old expectations for the new vision of positive health and responsibility for well-being.

For the most part, the discussions of primary care strategy omit recognition of (a) the "generalist" (doctor or nurse) in primary health care and (b) talk instead of pluralistic teams offering a wide range of services in the formal primary care sector. This decision begs the questions of personal care and the cost-effectiveness of health services without a generalist tier. Historically health services that are not protected from incremental specialist encroachment into the community become extremely expensive and fragmented at the point of delivery, the United States being a prime example.

Change of the order of magnitude proposed will demand a critical mass of health service staff who understand the virtues of uncertainty and the dangers of therapeutic dogma and who will question current practice and seek new ways to achieve justice in setting priorities. Indeed a basis for making choices in health service resource allocation is a prerequisite of informed give-and-take between scientists and politicians. Hence a rational research culture needs a structure for research and development that is easily understood and readily applied to biomedical, sociomedical, and health service studies. It must be relevant to molecular research, to tissue research, and to research on people in their community context or in population (public health) studies. The structure should clarify the relationships between projects, identify weaknesses in planning, and facilitate balanced development of work across a wide range of skills and objectives. Above all it must increase justice in research and development.

Developed by N. Stott and R. Pill, Figure 1.1 presents a research and development matrix that fulfills some of these criteria and provides a map that can be applied at any level in the human "systems cone" shown in Figure 1.2. Mapping helps clarify whether research is being conducted at an appropriate level and whether it is derived from a value-neutral, value-laden, or value-normative

Method	Disease Prevention	Treatment or Intervention	Health Promotion	Health Care Delivery
Development of new methods or techniques or basic science	A	B	C	D
Evaluation using current methods: Effectiveness, Quality, Cost of methods	E	F	G	H
Experimental introduction and evaluation	I	J	K	L
Research into uptake of changes and generalizability	M	N	O	P

Figure 1.1. Matrix of Research and Development

part of the systems cone. Prediction is easiest in value-neutral areas below the "person" level or when people are pooled to achieve normative (community) values. However, the values of individuals and families cannot be ignored in clinical decision making (McWhinney, 1989), and research is often most complex at the person level, where the doctor, the patient, and the illness all interact to influence outcome. The failure of successful dissemination of good research results is often due to failure to conduct research on the generalizability of specialist discoveries.

Examples of research activity have been chosen to illustrate application of the matrix in the context of the systems cone.

Development of New Methods, Techniques, or Basic Science

In the 1970s the Department of General Practice in Wales adopted a policy of research into common problems in family medicine.

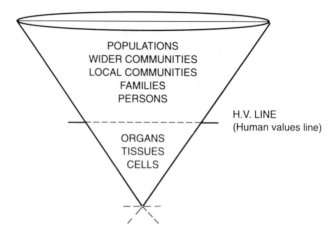

Figure 1.2. Human Systems Cone

For example, the department showed that 25% of consultations in an urban practice for simple upper respiratory infections were followed by a second consultation within 2 weeks for the same condition. Detailed analysis of this surprising statistic showed that the same clinical outcomes were obtained from high prescribers as low prescribers (Stott, 1979). In addition, it was found that reducing antibiotic or cough mixture prescribing made little difference to outcome in infants but did lead to fewer consultations for nonspecific upper respiratory infections in the 5- to 9-year-old group. The interplay between doctors' behavior and people's use of services led us on to research the results of communication skills teaching (Verby, Holden, & Davis, 1979), a review of the determinants of help-seeking behavior (Stott, 1983), and to research into health promotion and disease prevention. In terms of the matrix shown in Figure 1.1, we had moved from B and F to C and D.

During the 1980s a cohort of working-class families was studied by using qualitative and quantitative techniques to measure health behaviors (Pill & Stott, 1985; Stott & Pill, 1990b). This was "pure" research insofar as it represented a search to understand the reasons underlying mothers' health and life-style choices. One new research tool was developed: the Salience of Life-Style Index (Pill & Stott, 1987). Little evidence was found for a "general orientation to healthy life-styles" in the women studied. Instead preventive procedures (e.g., dental care or breast self-examination) and preventive practices (exercise, smoking cessation, alcohol intake, diet) seemed to be independent dimensions in the individuals concerned, with the possible exception of smoking and alcohol intake, which exhibited some correlation.

The same women also were studied longitudinally when an opportunity arose for a 5-year follow-up (Stott & Pill, 1990b). This work revealed little change in health behaviors in the cohort when quantitative scores were used. However, a complex picture was revealed when qualitative methods (individual and group interviews) were applied to the same subjects. This approach revealed that more than 50% of the women had been striving over the past 5 years to improve their own and their families' health against the odds of aging, family opposition to change, and the economic constraints of an urban life. We concluded that important findings had been diluted in the quantitative cohort data: that families can be trapped in a context that inhibits the adoption of healthful life-styles despite their attempts to change. This study represented a balance of quantitative and qualitative research techniques within matrix areas C and G (Figure 1.1). It also revealed how important it is for cohort research in primary care to be interpreted cautiously until information at the person/family level is also available (Figure 1.2).

Application of disciplined systems thinking to issues in family medicine can be illustrated further in the development of a risk-scoring system that predicts abnormal cervical smears. Wilkinson, Peters, Harvey, and Stott (1992) reviewed international, case-controlled studies to develop a risk scale based on independent factors of epidemiological importance. They then conducted a small-scale qualitative analysis of the acceptability of this scale to women in the sexually active age group, before applying it to 4,000 women prospectively at the time of their cervical smears. Encouraging results from this work make it tempting to promote the scale for wide-scale application. The research cycle will be incomplete, however, until the risk scale is tested again for predictive power and personal impact when applied to individuals in another population group, followed by an assessment of its generalizability and economic implications. In other words, an interplay between studies on populations and on individuals in the systems cone and between sectors A, E, I, and M in the research matrix provides a three-dimensional disciplined view of the research. Indeed the inadequacies of current cervical screening programs and their poor cost-effectiveness are a legacy of premature generalization of early research in the 1960s and 1970s, when longitudinal "natural history" studies still were considered to be ethical and randomized controlled trials to be feasible.

Evaluations Using Current Methods and Field Experiments

One of my most widely cited research studies is a double-blind, randomized, controlled trial investigating the treatment of middle respiratory infection (adults with cough and purulent sputum of up to 7 days duration, who were otherwise healthy) (Stott & West, 1976). More than 200 adults from three practices were randomized into antibiotic and placebo groups following an exercise to standardize the eliciting of chest signs by participating physicians. We found no significant difference in outcome when the groups were compared over the next 2 weeks. This work provided a useful null result (F in Figure 1.1), together with new data on the 14-day natural history of the condition (B in Figure 1.1).

Paradoxically, despite worldwide citations and confirmatory studies, there really has not been much evidence of change in clinical practice as a result of the new evidence (Stott, 1982). This paucity may have been partly due to the failure to progress the work at an early stage into further local studies with an evaluation of uptake/generalizability of the new ideas (J and N in the matrix).

Another possible reason for the failure to achieve general application of these results is the fact that the study dealt with a *group* of patients. In contrast, general practitioners deal with individuals in context, and it is well known that individual variables sometimes will override the best trial evidence on groups (McWhinney, 1989). Howie (1976) showed this clearly in his study of the management of sore throats, in which contextual variables influenced the choice of antibiotics to a major extent. Similarly Mulley (1990) showed that the scientific selection of treatment for prostatism can be influenced heavily by the fact that urodynamically superior suprapubic prostatectomy is more likely to cause ejaculation failure or impotence. This effect is quite unacceptable to some men but of little consequence to others. Human values, therefore, become a major variable in determining outcome: People need to be presented with readily understood data about personal risks, therapeutic options, and survival, rather than data about likely organ function alone. Our understanding of how to properly inform people about their choices in health care is still quite rudimentary and stands as an area for physician and nurse research.

The department's evaluation of health checks in general practice is a well-documented example of an evaluation of health care delivery in relation to disease prevention and health promotion (Stott & Pill, 1988). The department used the opportunity of an invitation for a "health check" that was sent to the patients of an inner-city practice in Cardiff to compare samples of people who did and did not respond to a first invitation. Transatlantic colleagues must realize that prior to 1990 the British public were quite unused to the concept of a *health check,* and so this research was an opportunity for a fresh understanding of people's choices before major political interference with the issues began.

Three categories of nonattenders were defined: those who refused the invitation, those who made but broke an appointment, and those who simply did not reply. These three groups differed in many respects and had different reasons for failing to attend, indicating the heterogeneity of nonresponders. The most important finding from this study, however, was that high-risk people were less likely to respond than low-risk people. The department concluded that an orchestrated cohort screening policy would be a very inefficient way to reach those at high risk, because so many low-risk individuals would need to be seen for each one at high risk (Pill & Stott, 1988). Morrell (1978) came to a similar conclusion after his London cohort screening study; Schwoon and Schmoll (1979) found that attenders for screening in Germany were likely to see the doctor more often, even when they did not feel ill; and D'Souza (1983) and Anderson (1984) came to similar conclusions. In terms of the matrix, the experimental introduction of a service (I, K, and L) did not support further work on its generalizability.

Unfortunately research often is ignored if it contradicts the prevailing political belief system. The U.K. Contract for family doctors in 1990 legislated for "registration health checks," "thrice-yearly health checks," and annual health checks for those over 75 years of age. Logical application and dissemination of research is, therefore, a major health policy issue (M, N, O, and P in Figure 1.1) because so few politicians have any grounding in scientific method and because management science is becoming a means to rationalize decision making based on unsatisfactory evidence. It is not unusual for managers to sneer at "purist attitudes in research"; they charge forward to make decisions on the best available evidence rather than through systematic evaluation of each step in the matrix.

Research Into Uptake

A major initiative to help family doctors and nurses regain a role in diabetic care was mounted in South Glamorgan in 1988 (Stott, Smail, & Peters, 1992). This development program involved training many practice nurses in diabetic care, providing continuing medical education opportunities, campaigning to improve chiropody and dietetic services, and setting up an auditing mechanism to monitor standards. A nurse facilitator visited each practice to kindle active involvement during the development phase, and a clerk with a laptop computer visited each participating family practice annually to extract items reflecting the standards from the clinical records of all diabetic patients. The family doctors received a printout that showed their own pattern of care compared with pooled area norms.

More than 50% of practices in South Glamorgan enrolled in the scheme during the first 2 years, and the 1991 quality control audit showed that the standard of care was quite high. Data from more than 2,000 diabetic people are now available for interpractice comparisons (unattributed data) and for year-on-year intrapractice performance analysis. These data can be presented as individual trends over time, pooled cross-sectional practice data, or local community data. The hypothesis growing from this peer review process (J, K, L in Figure 1.1) is that it will lead, within 3 years, to realistic clinical targets for diabetic care.

The next stage will be to see how generalizable the diabetic project is farther afield, to see whether standards can be maintained at reasonable cost, and to compare efficiency and effectiveness when compared with a specialist-dominated system of outpatient care.

Target setting is one possible mechanism to stimulate innovation, as well as to goad those who are reluctant to respond to the calls for change. However, the results of current enthusiasm for target setting remain to be proven. Family doctors need to monitor the adverse effects of national target setting because it is at the doctor-patient interface that the tensions between individual and community needs are felt most acutely. For example, the national target on smoking loses its priority in the face of an individual's grief, or the importance of screening a person's blood pressure wanes into insignificance when the family is in crisis. Family medicine overflows with individual reasons for default from cross-sectional population targets, and crude statistical returns are insensitive to such detail. If a target for payment is 90% coverage, then 89% is failure; nothing is more exasperating than finding that human concern and compassion at the individual level have been turned sour by penalties at the population level.

The systems cone shown in Figure 1.2 is becoming an important conceptual construct for negotiations with politicians/planners because it can be used or abused as it highlights the interrelationships between personal and population medicine. The issues have ethical, practical, and financial implications for family doctors in the 1990s because political decisions are taken for populations, whereas the consequential actions have to be applied to individuals. Our experience in the United Kingdom is that politicians have little concern or insight into the clinicians' dilemmas, and specialists often assume generalizability of their research results without wider evaluation from those who work in generalist contexts.

Research in Family Medicine:
Pure or Applied?

Family physicians' biomedical and social science backgrounds draw them naturally into the upper left sectors of the matrix (Figure

1.1), whereas the new calls for health promotion and efficient health service delivery draw them down into the lower right-hand sectors.

This is not a "pure" and "applied" division, but it does reaffirm the dual motives behind the scientific process: to understand the natural world and to control it. Mapping research into the matrix helps kindle a more balanced view of research output and sets primary care research into a wider perspective.

The serious academic in family medicine still will be dismayed by the way some health service reforms are introduced despite opposing evidence. To try to control the natural world seems to be a hallmark of the politician more than of the scientist. The hallmark of the true scientist must be to *understand* the natural world and to evaluate properly the risk of systematic and random errors during the introduction of new technologies.

When research involves many encounters with ill and well people in context, rather than with diseases, the integration of qualitative and quantitative methods is desirable. A quantitative study in which individual or family values are important variables may miss the point unless enriched with a qualitative arm (Stott & Pill, 1990a). The close integration of qualitative and quantitative research methods is beginning to look like a hallmark for research and development in family medicine. Population data then can be evaluated without losing the rich understanding that comes from the study of individuals. A suitable strategy would be to approach any R & D issue in this dualistic way. Our tactics are likely to involve an interdisciplinary approach to research, and "creative tension" will be one (desirable) outcome from the marriage.

Conclusion

The discipline of primary health care has much to do with being in close touch with the community served. Pragmatism and commitment, however, are not enough; there is also an urgent need to relate all research to core theory/constructs. Application of systems thinking and the research matrix to all studies should assist in maintaining such a perspective, as well as in highlighting a hallmark of primary care research: the combined use of qualitative and quantitative methodologies at every level. In addition, the lure of purely descriptive work should be eschewed in the 1990s. It is nearly always possible to test a hypothesis or conduct an experiment with the descriptive (inductive) element flowing naturally from both processes.

References

Anderson, R. (1984). Health promotion: An overview. *European Monographs in Health Education Research, 6*, 1-76.

D'Souza, M. (1983). The case against a medical check-up. In J. Fry (Ed.), *Common dilemmas in family medicine* (pp. 322-336). Lancaster: MTP.

Howie, J. C. R. (1976). Clinical judgment and antibiotic use in general practice. *British Medical Journal, 2*, 1061-1064.

McWhinney, I. R. (1989). *A textbook of family medicine.* New York: Oxford University Press.

Morrell, D. (1978). Screening in general practice. *Health Trends, 10*, 40-41.

Mulley, A. G. (1990). Medical decision-making and practice variation. In T. Anderson & G. Mooney (Eds.), *The challenges of medical practice variations* (pp. 59-75). Basingstoke: Macmillan.

Pill, R. M., & Stott, N. C. H. (1985). Preventive procedures and practices among working class women: New data and fresh insights. *Social Science and Medicine, 21*, 975-983.

Pill, R. M., & Stott, N. C. H. (1987). Development of a measure of potential health behavior: A salience of life-style index. *Social Science and Medicine, 24*, 125-134.

Pill, R. M., & Stott, N. C. H. (1988). Invitation to attend a health check in a general practice setting. *Journal of the Royal College of General Practitioners, 38*, 57-60.

Schwoon, D. R., & Schmoll, H. J. (1979). Motivation to participate in cancer screening programmes. *Social Science and Medicine, 13a*, 283-286.

Snow, C. P. (1964). *Two cultures: And a second look.* New York: Cambridge University Press.

Stott, N. C. H. (1979). Management and outcome of winter upper respiratory infections in children. *British Medical Journal, 1*, 29-31.

Stott, N. C. H. (1982). Clinical trial in general practice. *British Medical Journal, 285*, 941-944.

Stott, N. C. H. (1983). Help seeking: How, where, why, whither? *Primary health care: Bridging the gap between theory and practice* (Vol. 4, pp. 33-56). New York: Springer Verlag.

Stott, N. C. H., & Pill, R. M. (1988). *Health checks in general practice: Why some people attend and others do not.* Cardiff: University of Wales College of Medicine.

Stott, N. C. H., & Pill, R. M. (1990a). Advice yes, dictate no: Patients' views on health promotion in the consultation. *Family Practice, 7*(2), 125-131.

Stott, N. C. H., & Pill, R. M. (1990b). *Making changes: A study of working-class mothers and changes made in their health-related behavior over 5 years.* Cardiff: University of Wales College of Medicine.

Stott, N. C. H., Smail, J., & Peters, J. (1992). *Enhanced care of people with diabetes in South Glamorgan.* Cardiff: University of Wales College of Medicine.

Stott, N. C. H., & West, R. R. (1976). Double-blind randomized controlled trial: Antibiotics in patients with cough and purulent sputum. *British Medical Journal, 2,* 556-559.

Verby, J., Holden, P., & Davis, R. H. (1979). Peer review of consultations in primary care: Use of audiovisual recordings. *British Medical Journal, 1,* 1686-1688.

Wilkinson, C. E., Peters, T. J., Harvey, I. M., & Stott, N. C. H. (1992). Risk targeting in cervical screening: A new look at an old problem. *British Journal of General Practice, 42,* 435-438.

World Health Organization. (1978). *Primary health care: Report of the international conference.* Geneva: Author.

2 How Can Quality Research Be Done in Primary Care Practice?

CAROL P. HERBERT

Empowerment is a catchword that emerged from political movements of the last two decades. It describes the process by which groups who feel powerless develop a sense of self-efficacy and take control of their lives. Empowerment requires (a) a *predisposing* belief that change is possible, (b) a set of *enabling* skills, and (c) an environment that responds to and *reinforces* changed behavior.

In this chapter I describe the process of empowerment of primary care practitioners to conduct quality research. I define "quality research in primary care practice"; identify predisposing, enabling, and reinforcing factors for doing such research; and describe some existing environments that represent successful examples.

Defining Quality Research

All research must begin with an accurate operational definition of a question. My question is, How can quality research be done in primary care practice? Let us go through the steps of refining and operationalizing the question by using the *Random House Dictionary* (1987) as our resource.

Quality has many definitions, but in this context the most applicable are "high grade of superiority, excellence" and "marked by a concentrated expenditure of involvement, concern or commitment" (p. 1579). The research endeavor of interest here must be characterized both by excellence and by involvement, concern, and commitment.

Primary care refers to "medical care by a physician or other health care professional who is the patient's first contact with and who provides access to the health care system" (p. 1537).

Clearly it matters whether we mean primary health care or primary medical care when we consider how to and who shall do quality research. For purposes of maximum generalizability, I suggest we are interested in the former and in the sense of functionally defining it according to the work, rather than by the discipline of the worker. Thus, for example, primary health care could involve urban street workers, physicians' assistants, and native health care workers, along with physicians and nurses.

Practice is defined as "the business of a professional person" (p. 1517) and can take place in the office, the home, the hospital, or other community settings such as schools, family planning clinics, and health units. This broad definition is critical in considering "primary care practice" because first contact includes, but is not limited to, the office setting.

Finally what is meant by *research?* A simple definition is the systematic collection of data in order to shed light on an unanswered question. For research to take place, there must be both a question to be answered (Armstrong, Calnan, & Grace, 1990) and a system for knowledge acquisition and recording.

What constitutes a relevant question depends very much on the observer's viewpoint. Much energy has been expended on the development of research agendas for primary care and for family medicine (Herbert, 1991; Seifert, 1982; Shank, 1980). Some of these agendas have been little more than lists, while others have attempted to establish a taxonomy and/or hierarchy of questions. Most agendas reflect the belief that groups of university-based researchers can and should a priori define what will be acceptable research questions. Few attempts at agenda setting involve the community—either that of patients or of practitioners—in setting questions. This scarcity has resulted in suspicion and cynicism about the quality of research in primary care practice, both in terms of intrinsic value and applicability.

It is the contention here that quality research in primary care practice requires both that the research be *action oriented* (that changed practice is the desired outcome) and that the questions *take into account the needs of the community.* As Seifert (1991) noted, "The truth of the matter is, patients, practitioner-researchers, laboratory practices and community boards are not optional!" (p. 4).

Three other criteria can be applied to any research question:

1. The question must be important to the researcher.
2. The question must be answerable in the available time and with the available resources.
3. The researcher must be able to fit the question, large or small, into an organizing research framework, such as that described by Stott in Chapter 1 of this volume.

Unfortunately our specialist colleagues sometimes considered primary care research questions to be trivial, uninteresting, or unimportant. This attitude has affected researchers both in the grant application process and when papers are submitted for peer review. A promising development in changing this trend is the recent formation of the Agency for Health Care Policy and Research (AHCPR) by the National Institutes of Health, which recognizes the importance of research questions dealing with problems that are common, costly, cause morbidity, and affect people's self-esteem and their activities of daily living (Mayfield & Grady, 1991).

To understand our defined question better, then, let us restate it: How can excellent, involved, and committed systematic data collection to shed light on an unanswered question with the ultimate goal of changing practice be conducted at the level of first contact of individuals, families, and communities with the health care system in office, home, hospital, or other settings?

Predisposing and Enabling Factors

A historical example may help clarify some of the necessary predisposing and enabling factors for carrying out primary care research as defined here. A Scottish general practitioner at the turn of the century, James Mackenzie, endeavored to understand heart function by careful observation and recording during 15 years and succeeded in delineating sinus arrhythmia (Mair, 1973). His key *predisposing* factors were (a) a belief that his observations were important and worthwhile, (b) a curious mind, and (c) persistence. His research was *enabled* by an organized recording system (by hand, no computers) and by his personal control of the practice environment as a solo practitioner. *Reinforcing* factors did not include professional advancement, fame, money, or social status—indeed, on the basis of short-term productivity, Mackenzie never would have achieved tenure in a medical school. His reinforcement came from the pure intellectual pleasure of answering a self-posed question and his unwavering belief that patient care might be improved by his work.

Some things have changed during the decades; others have not. Key predisposing factors for individuals continue to be curiosity, a sense of self-worth, patience, a belief in the importance of one's work, and meticulousness in recording what is seen or heard. Quality research still can be driven purely by individual vision. In a publish-or-perish institutional environment, however, it may be that quantity wins out over quality. At the same time, communities increasingly—and appropriately—want a say in the research agenda. Moreover, the questions we now are asking often require more cases than a single provider can collect in a reasonable period of time. Thus a belief in the advantage and necessity of collaboration, both in developing the research design and in data collection, has become necessary for many practice questions.

Enabling factors include the practical aspects of (a) organizing one or more practice settings for research, (b) identifying research questions of importance to the community, (c) recruiting and retaining subjects, and (d) developing collaborative teams where necessary. Networking of practices has enabled the development and conduct of research that never could have been done by individuals. Networks may be local, regional, national, or international, and they may be university based, project based, or organization/discipline based. Notable examples include the Thames Valley Family Practice Research Unit, the fledgling Family Practice Research Network in British Columbia, and the Ambulatory Sentinel Practice Network (ASPN), all described below. Other examples are the Canadian National Research System (Report of the Working Group on the National Recording System, 1988) and the International Primary Care Network (IPCN) (Culpepper & Froom, 1988).

One can construct a hierarchy of possible relationships between research partners, which I have termed the "7-*c's* of research relationship." These are cooperation, coordination, collaboration, convincing, co-opting, coercion, and collusion. I contend that what we are aiming for is a mix between cooperation and collaboration. Four examples of such facilitative research environments are considered below.

Examples of Empowerment in Primary Care Research

THAMES VALLEY FAMILY PRACTICE RESEARCH UNIT

The Thames Valley Family Practice Research Unit (1991) is an example of collaboration between a research-oriented university department of family medicine and local community physicians with an interest in research. The unit provides the infrastructure for a partnership between the Centre for Studies in Family Medicine at The University of Western Ontario, and the London Chapter of the College of Family Physicians of Canada, and is funded for an initial 5-year period (1989-1994) by the Ontario Ministry of Health. The unit's goal is to focus on issues relevant to family practice with a view to improving health care for the population by enhancing the quality and efficiency of service provided by family physicians.

The unit has set the following action-oriented research agenda:

1 Identifying the problems of caring for *disadvantaged groups*
2. Providing better coordinated and enhanced *home-based care* for the elderly and chronically ill
3. Improving *preventive care* in the family physician's office for immunization, screening, and life-style modification
4. Improving *communication* between family physicians and specialists, other health professionals, and patients
5. Developing appropriate *research methods* for conducting studies in family practice

After 2 years the success of this model can be measured by its research output: 7 research grants and 6 additional studies undertaken with unit resources, 18 peer-reviewed publications and 22 columns, and 10 current projects and 11 proposed projects. What have been the key elements in this endeavor? First, sufficient funding was provided for an infrastructure to support less-experienced researchers. Second, the unit built on the research experience of a mature department of family medicine with a critical mass of trained primary care researchers and a record of success in grants, studies, and publications. Third, the organizers fundamentally believed in the value of partnership between university and community and included a community physician who was funded to act part-time as a liaison between the two partners. Previous research by the center has proven that well-organized projects can be carried out in family physicians' offices. The Thames Valley Family Practice Research Unit represents the natural extension of that experience.

B.C. FAMILY PRACTICE RESEARCH NETWORK PROJECT

A second example of developing collaboration between academic and community physicians is the Family Practice Research Network (FPRN) project of the University of British Columbia (Herbert, 1990). Begun in February 1991, this project aims to develop a self-sustaining research infrastructure to facilitate primary care research in communities across the province.

During the past few years, community-based faculty have observed and participated in research carried out by second-year residents who must complete a mandatory project. Projects have been innovative and practical, fueling the interest of their community preceptors in the research process. Skepticism remains: Research is feared to be time-consuming, costly, difficult, or interfering with confidentiality of records. However, an increasing number of community-based faculty have stated an interest in becoming involved in research, expressing a desire for training in research methods and a need for advice and support in grant writing, proposal development, and writing for publication.

Despite very limited funding, the FPRN project is off and running, with the following stated goals:

1. To assist community-based family physicians and other primary care providers to develop research skills

2. To create a computerized system to allow data collection from family practice teaching sites in B.C.
3. To provide access to information and consultation from remote sites that are part of the Rural and Remote Residency Training Program

During the first year, we targeted two practice settings for data collection and networking: the Queen Charlotte Islands, which is a Rural and Remote Residency Training site, and our newly established Regional Family Practice Residency Program in Chilliwack, a small community about 60 miles from Vancouver.

We have provided consultation and mentorship to the six community physicians serving the Queen Charlotte Islands (population 6,000), with the resultant submission of five letters of intent from these physicians to a research foundation on native health issues. Two projects received grants for the development of full proposals: one on Pap smear screening and the other on diabetes education. Project teams were constituted as university/community partnerships, with full involvement at all stages of native health workers and members of the native community. Both proposals have involved intensive collaboration, including an initial site visit by the university participants, developmental work within the community by the local physicians, a university-based workshop, and collaborative writing and editing.

The Pap smear project is a particularly good example of community-based action research. This project grew out of a survey carried out by Dr. Betty Calam (Calam, Bass, & Deagle, 1992) that identified differential cervical screening rates between Haida and non-Haida women. Attempts to discover why this difference existed have resulted in increased interest within the native community in providing alternative opportunities for preventive care that take native experience into account. The research design includes an optimal blending of quantitative measures of outcome and qualitative analysis of the experience of individuals. It is hoped that it will be a prototype for other culturally sensitive preventive/health promotion services.

In Chilliwack we have developed a pilot project to computerlink four office sites to the regional hospital for data acquisition on the experience of the residents and to provide them with computer access to a librarian and CD-ROM. The result has been a 300% increase in use of library services. Regular meetings of the project team in Chilliwack have been critical for team building.

Again the central theme of the network project is empowerment of practice-based physicians to ask answerable research questions in their own settings. It does this by respecting their competence and intellect and by recognizing that skills can be taught to willing learners. At the same time, the necessity of integration of research in the practical reality of daily work is being recognized. Consequently the project is proceeding slowly, carefully, and organically, evolving according to the experience of the participants.

COLLABORATION WITH THE DEVELOPING WORLD

In an international context, the College of Family Physicians of Canada undertook an innovative and exciting experiment in 1989 to encourage primary care research in developing countries. In a Canadian-government-sponsored project entitled "Does the Family Medicine Paradigm Have Relevance in the Developing World?" (Grava-Gubins et al., 1990), a group of 14 primary care physicians from 13 countries came to Singapore to meet for one intensive week with five Canadian family physicians who acted as advisors in helping them write their own research proposals. These proposals were designed to be funded, completed, and reported on at the WONCA Scientific Assembly held in Vancouver, B.C., in 1992. Only two of the 14 participants had some limited prior research experience; the rest were interested novices.

By the end of the week, all proposals were well under way, and, as of this writing, 10 participants have already successfully completed their projects.

When we described the planned project to epidemiologist colleagues in 1989, we were met with skepticism. How could practicing physicians without research training write research proposals, let alone carry them out? Indeed it is likely that only family doctors would have had the temerity to attempt such a task. Was this an example of our limited understanding of the complexity of the endeavor? In fact, analogous to clinical problem solving in the primary care setting, both the Canadian and the international participants understood our limitations but built on our strengths. We negotiated the statement of questions so that they became answerable in the context of the questioner. We listed the resources necessary for project completion, providing literature searches on site and ongoing advice by mail and by fax over many months. Above all, we respected one another as capable and committed health care workers who could master problem-solving skills and learn from one another.

AMBULATORY SENTINEL PRACTICE NETWORK

Primary care practice-based research networks are not a new idea: Groups in Australia, France, Canada, New Zealand, and the United Kingdom have used them to gather data on a variety of clinical questions. Such networks ameliorate the difficulties of generalizability in single practice studies and of insufficient patients for study. Since 1970, the Dutch sentinel stations have investigated approximately 60 topics (Green & Lutz, 1990). NaReS, the Canadian National Research System (Report of the Working Group on the National Recording System, 1988), has carried out a variety of studies since the early 1970s, when the network was first developed for influenza surveillance.

The Ambulatory Sentinel Practice Network (ASPN) (Hickner, 1991) illustrates the principles underlying a truly successful practice-based network. The concept first was presented at the 1979 meeting of the North American Primary Care Research Group (NAPCRG). Funding was obtained from NAPCRG and the Rockefeller Foundation, and data collection began in 1982.

The network is centered in Denver, Colorado, because of the strong support of Dr. Larry Green and the University of Colorado Department of Family Medicine there. From an initial membership of 38 practices, it has grown to include 71 practices and 334 practitioners in Canada and the United States. Few have dropped out; those who have, have cited time as the major drawback (Green, Niebauer, Miller, & Lutz, 1991).

Although ideas for studies can originate anywhere, the majority have come from practitioners, with all requiring the approval of the board of directors. Explicit guidelines have been stated (Green et al., 1984). Studies must

1. Be relevant to the well-being of patients or primary care providers
2. Have strict criteria that can be formulated

3. Not be too time-consuming for the practices
4. Encourage practice participation
5. Be of adequate importance to attract funding
6. Have a study question more appropriately addressed by a large network study
7. Have an identified principal investigator.

In addition, the following "relative guidelines" recommend that studies

1. Have potential for impact on public policy
2. Have potential for impact on development of research in primary care
3. Build on existing knowledge or address a knowledge vacuum
4. Can combine psychological and biomedical questions for the same subject.

From 1982 to 1991, ASPN studied spontaneous abortion, headache, pelvic inflammatory disease, herpes, chest pain, type II diabetes mellitus, low back pain, CT scan for investigation of headache, falls, depression, carpal tunnel syndrome, cough, and HIV seroprevalence.

ASPN is a financially and administratively independent organization with a full-time physician-director, executive director, research coordinator, and secretary. This administrative structure, evolved by trial and error, is necessary to operate a large, geographically dispersed primary care network. The strength of ASPN, however, is its practice base, with studies either originating from practitioners or supported and approved by them, despite the time and effort required to obtain consensus.

Conclusion

The examples given in this chapter demonstrate the principles of empowerment of quality research in the primary care practice.

Predisposing factors in all situations included willing and interested community-based physicians and committed, experienced academic researchers, with all collaborators believing in the intrinsic value of shared power. Egalitarian relationships require continuous effort to ensure that goals are derived by consensus and that knowledge is returned to participants for their own use. Individuals must understand their strengths and limitations and must know how to ask a research question that is answerable within the constraints of available time and resources or, alternatively, how to extend those resources by collaboration in research teams and by obtaining external funding. Above all, participants must believe that health policy and clinical practice can be changed by practice-derived knowledge.

Enabling factors include:

1. Sufficient funding for an infrastructure to provide research workshops, materials, fellowships, advice, and mentorship
2. Education and experience in research skills during residency training
3. Organization of projects to minimize practice disruption (learning from our past mistakes)
4. Increased funding for research in primary care practice
5. Development of methods that are suited to primary care research questions, including the collaborative research process itself
6. Primary care research networks—local, regional, national, and international. Some networks allow "painless participation" in quality research with expert advice available centrally, while others actively foster community-based researchers.

Reinforcing factors include successful attainment of grants, recognition by peers at research forums where work in progress can be presented for constructive criticism, regional and national primary care meetings for sharing of research questions and results with like-minded colleagues from both "gown" and "town" settings, publication of results in peer-reviewed journals, and faculty appointments and promotion within the ranks. Most reinforcing of all is the experience of change in clinical practice or health policy based on knowledge obtained through research.

The use of results by the communities from which information has been obtained is the true measure of "quality research in primary care practice," whether it be the community of practitioners, the community of patients, or the larger political community.

26   GENERAL ISSUES

References

Armstrong, D., Calnan, M., & Grace, J. (1990). *Research methods for general practitioners.* Oxford, UK: Oxford University Press.

Calam, B., Bass, M. J., & Deagle, G. (1992). Pap smear screening rates: Coverage on the southern Queen Charlotte Islands. *Canadian Family Physician, 38*(5), 1103-1109.

Culpepper, L., & Froom, J. (1988). The international primary care network: Purposes, methods, and policies. A report from ASPN. *Family Medicine, 20,* 197-201.

Grava-Gubins, I., Hennen, B., Elmslie, T. T., Herbert, C. P., Labrecque, M., & Maclachlan, R. (1990). Does the family medicine paradigm have relevance in the developing world? [Abstract]. *Canadian Family Physician, 36,* 2172-2174.

Green, L. A., & Lutz, L. J. (1990). Notions about networks: Primary care practices in pursuit of improved primary care. In J. Mayfield & M. L. Grady (Eds.), *Primary care research: An agenda for the 90's* (pp. 120-125). Rockville, MD: Agency for Health Care Policy and Research.

Green, L., Niebauer, L. J., Miller, R. S., & Lutz, L. J. (1991). An analysis of reasons for discontinuing participation in a practice-based research network. *Family Medicine, 23*(6), 447-449.

Green, L. A., Wood, M., Becker, L. A., Farley, E. S., Freeman, W. L., Froom, J., Hames, C., Niebauer, L. J., Rosser, W. W., & Siefert, M. (1984). The Ambulatory Sentinel Practice Network: Purposes, methods and policies. *Journal of Family Practice, 18,* 275-280.

Herbert, C. P. (1990). *Family practice research network.* Unpublished research proposal.

Herbert, C. P. (1991). Why family practice research? *Canadian Family Physician, 37,* 335-338.

Hickner, J. (1991). Practice-based primary care research networks. In H. Hibbard, P. A. Nutting, & M. L. Grady (Eds.), *Primary care research: Theory and methods* (pp. 13-22). Rockville, MD: Agency for Health Care Policy and Research.

Mair, A. (1973). *Sir James Mackenzie, M.D., general practitioner, 1853-1925.* Edinburgh: Churchill, Livingstone.

Mayfield, J., & Grady, M. L. (Eds.). (1990). *Primary care research: An agenda for the 90's.* Rockville, MD: Agency for Health Care Policy and Research.

Random House Dictionary of the English Language (2nd ed., unabridged). (1987). New York: Random House.

Report of the Working Group on the National Recording System. (1988, March). Report presented to the National Research Committee of the College of Family Physicians of Canada, Toronto, Ontario.

Seifert, M. (1982). Research in family practice: A blueprint for the eighties. *Family Practice Research Journal, 1*(4), 211-223.

Seifert, M. (1991). *The NAPCRG Working Group for Strategic Planning—A practitioner's response.* Unpublished manuscript.

Shank, C. J. (1980). A taxonomy for research. *Family Medicine Teacher, 12*(5), 22-23.

Thames Valley Family Practice Research Unit. (1991). *Two year report.* London, Ontario: The University of Western Ontario, Centre for Studies in Family Medicine.

3 Ethical Issues in Primary Care Research

BRIAN HENNEN

Getting involved in primary care research enables practitioners to understand and be better at what they do. How one ought to conduct that research, all possible things considered, constitutes its ethics.

Patients' perceptions of health and illness extend far beyond what most health care professionals learn about in the usual health science school curriculum. Today's concepts of health include a sense of well-being and self-determination. Illness, on the other hand, is an experience of several dimensions. Cassell (1976) emphasized four: (a) loss of control, (b) loss of a sense of omnipotence, (c) loss of connectedness, and (d) loss of the power of reason. These perceptions lead directly to a number of ethical considerations. Issues of autonomy of the patient, confidentiality of information, truthfulness and control of the information available to patients, paternalistic behavior by health professionals, and consent by patients for interventions taken in their lives are all profoundly implicated in determining how we ought to behave as providers and as researchers.

In clinical work, *patient-centered care* requires the provider to develop with the patient a mutual understanding of the latter's problems that reflects both of their perspectives. It includes helping the patient reveal the personal story of his or her illness, determining a common ground of understanding about that illness, and agreeing on management strategies acceptable to both parties (Weston, Brown, & Stewart, 1989). In primary care research, the ethics involve fundamentally these same personal relationships.

27

A Historical Perspective

The story of modern ethical guidelines for medical research may begin with the two basic principles of the 1948 Nuremberg Code: Subjection to experimentation must be totally voluntary, and the research subject should be fully informed in advance about the procedure and its hazards. Sixteen years later, the World Medical Association's Declaration of Helsinki distinguished between nontherapeutic clinical research (for which the Nuremberg rules stand) and "clinical research combined with professional care," in which the doctor may combine research and care only to the extent that the former is justified by its therapeutic value for the patient (Beauchamp & Childress, 1979).

In 1966 the National Institutes of Health in the United States developed policies and procedures for ethics review of research protocols based on three basic guidelines: (a) protection of the rights and welfare of the individual, (b) judgment on the method used to obtain informed consent, and (c) determination of the risks and potential benefits of the investigation (Frankel, 1972). These guidelines are today the basis of the ethical review of protocols required by the College of Family Physicians of Canada through its National Research Committee (Lewis et al., 1988). The Public Health Service of the U.S. Department of Health, Education and Welfare established a set of guidelines in 1969 for the "protection of the individual as a research subject" (Public Health Service, 1969). With a similar goal, the Medical Research Council of Canada (1987) produced the *Guidelines on Research Involving Human Subjects* (these guidelines currently are applied to ethical review of research studies in my own setting, The University of Western Ontario). Because primary medical care research almost always employs human subjects or their records or specimens, similar standards must apply to it.

Research in primary health care is relatively recent. In Britain, research in general practice actually predates university acceptance of its disciplinary status, early work by Mackenzie (1917) and Pickles (1939) being outstanding examples.

As the primary care academic disciplines have matured quickly in recent times, so also have the ethical standards of research. What was acceptable only a few years ago is no longer. Relatively recent academic writings on general practice research had little

or no mention of ethics (Eimerl & Laidlaw, 1969; Watson, 1982).
One writer on medical surveys and clinical trials actually argued:

> If there is evidence that a new treatment may be safe and effective,
> if there is reason to think that it is an improvement on existing ones,
> and if controls are given a good established treatment, there can be
> no ethical or legal objections against a clinical trial, no matter whether
> it is blind or otherwise, and the patients' consent is as unnecessary
> as if an investigation was carried out on their case records. (Glaser,
> 1964, p. 116)

Today's ethics do not countenance clinical trials without consent,
nor do they encourage the curious perusal of patient records,
however scientific the intent, without consent. The same author
suggested that distinctions between severe disease with uncertain treatment efficacy and disease that is mild or for which there
is effective treatment could determine the degree of patient understanding and consent required to be solicited before undertaking clinical trials. Today's standards of ethics do not so freely
allow a different standard of disclosure to be applied according
to intervention risk or treatability of conditions.

Qualitative researchers conducting ethnographic studies have
guidelines such as the Principles of Professional Responsibility
of the American Anthropological Association. These include (a)
actively working to safeguard informants' rights, interests, and
sensitivities, (b) communicating the research objectives clearly to
them, (c) protecting their privacy, (d) not exploiting them, and (e)
making reports of studies available to them (Spradley, 1980).

The hospital setting has been predominant as a site for clinical
research. When considering research on subjects' records or specimens, we find some guidelines in hospital board rules set out in
public legislation. For example, "a hospital Board may permit a
member of the medical staff, but only for scientific research that
has been approved by the medical staff Advisory Committee, to
inspect and receive information from a medical record and to be
given copies therefrom" (p. 498). Such information is not to be
used "for any purpose other than the purposes of compiling statistics and carrying out medical and epidemiological research for
or approved by the Department and the Commission" (Revised

Regulations of Ontario, 1970, p. 498). But what ethical guidelines pertain to community-based primary care practice?

The Community Context and the Nature of Primary Care Research

Because primary care disciplines deal with a mix of clinical medicine, social problems, wellness, preventive maneuvers, health education, and families as patients, the kinds of research that a primary health care provider might undertake are wide ranging. And primary care involves many sites: office, hospital, home, and nursing home. Howie (1979) divided research studies in primary care according to site, content, and methodology.

In considering some of the differences faced by primary health care researchers compared with other fields, Coulehan, Shaffner, and Block (1985) characterized primary medical practice research: It is based on ordinary medical practice. The investigator is more likely to be the personal physician. Studies deal with common problems. The research has different end points of study completion. It is more likely to deal with the process than the content of practice. It is inextricably tied into the patient-doctor relationship. It has a high incidence of psychosocial aspects. It is more likely to be multidisciplinary and to have a qualitative component.

As the primary health care disciplines develop more qualitative research methods to complement the more usual quantitative ones, the research menu becomes even more extensive. It follows that the ethics of that research also has to be wide ranging and extensive.

The Major Concerns

In primary care research, Howie (1979) considered the first major ethical issue to be one of conflict of the "therapeutic imperative" (Coulehan et al., 1985) of the physician providing care to the individual versus the collective ethic of research on numbers of people to contribute to the general welfare. The second main issue he addressed is the conflict between the healer's power position (the coercive potential of the personal physician in inviting patients to take part in studies) versus the autonomy and freely informed consent of patients to choose to take part.

Coulehan et al. (1985) elaborated on these issues, saying that the physician

> must avoid using his therapeutic relationship to persuade a patient to participate. . . . If the physician has a warranted (not idiosyncratic) belief that one treatment in a trial is more efficacious or more appropriate for that type of patient than another, it would be unethical for him to undertake the trial. (pp. 220-221)

This decision requires a consideration of what some call "equipoise," which is a state of genuine uncertainty on the part of the clinical investigator regarding the comparative therapeutic merits of each arm in a trial (Freedman, 1987). What Coulehan et al. (1985) were saying is, no equipoise, no study; also "however small the risks, a clinical trial is *not* ordinary medical care and must be considered a temporary, partial suspension of the therapeutic imperative" (p. 221). In considering a physician's duty to society, Veatch (1990) went further: "There is no moral permission to engage in behaviors such as research, public health and public policy activities that do not directly benefit the patient" (p. 292). In other words, we cannot assume a professional mandate to engage in these activities without public consultation or individual consent.

Exceptions Prove the Rule

In clinical medicine, guidelines often are violated when exceptions are found necessary by a physician who has taken into account the individual patient's particular problem and the context in which the problem presents. In ethics, too, exceptions to the rules may be found. Ashworth (1981), for example, would allow exemptions from the consent requirement for ethical issues of research when educational practices and tests were involved or where the signed consent of a patient is the only record linking the subject to the research and the study is one in which breach of confidentiality was the principal risk involved. (The current debate over anonymous HIV testing is an example of where signed consent may be inappropriate in certain potential research projects.)

Should the Research Be Done at All?

Shaffer (1972) wrote: "Perhaps the most basic question of all from the moral-ethical standpoint is whether certain lines of research, despite their promise of exciting discoveries about the nature of life, should even be pursued at all" (p. 4). Lynch (1990), in a discussion with others, considered whether terminally ill patients should be asked to take part in randomized controlled studies. Some discussants rejected the proposition outright, particularly for trials involving a nontreatment or placebo control. Others argued that such patients may be asked to participate if they gave their consent and if it is clear that no other kinds of subjects are suitable to determine the expected outcome of the study. Although still relatively infrequent in primary care, randomized control studies may become more common in light of the increased interest for pharmaceutical studies in primary care settings (see Hilditch, Chapter 11, this volume).

Hellman and Hellman (1991) presented one side of an excellent debate on randomized controlled trials, arguing that "researchers participating in such studies are required to modify their ethical commitments to individual patients and do serious damage to the concept of the physician as a practising, empathetic professional who is primarily concerned with each patient as an individual" (p. 1585). In contrast, Pasamani (1991) argued that "there is potential conflict between the roles of physician and physician scientist, and for this reason society has created mechanisms to ensure that the interests of individual patients are served should they elect to participate in a clinical trial" (p. 1589). He concluded, "Properly carried out, with informed consent, clinical equipoise and a design adequate to answer the questions posed, randomized clinical trials protect physicians and their patients from therapies that are ineffective or toxic" (p. 1589). Pasamani argued that, without randomized controlled trials, we would fall back into a dependency on physicians' hunches, which, in the past, frequently have been proven incorrect. He set out the general features that must be part of properly designed trials, including informed consent, equipoise, the availability of a data-monitoring committee to stop the trial if the accumulating data destroy the state of equipoise, a well-designed critical test of the therapeutic alternatives with appropriate statistical analysis, and the trial having a good chance of settling an open question.

Increased Vulnerability

As patient advocate, the primary care practitioner must be particularly vigilant when vulnerable subjects are about to be involved in research. Vulnerable subjects or patients may include the incompetent (very young or cognitively impaired), those who come from debilitating environments, those who have coercive-dependent relationships, those who have minority group status, those whose medical condition makes them incapable of self-determination, and the poor who might participate for financial reward. Meslin and Lowy (1990) noted that the potential costs to research subjects include inconvenience, financial cost, anxiety, pain, and permanent harm. In this volume, Farley (Chapter 5) addresses the ethical recruitment of subjects for research, and Freeman, Gelberg, and Mehr discuss the vulnerability of Natives, the homeless, and the institutional elderly in Chapters 14, 15, and 17, respectively.

Sex Bias and Inadequate Representation in Studies

Recent reviews of current medical research publications have pointed out significant sex bias. Cohen (1991) cited a review of leading medical journals reporting many examples of such bias, categorized into four types: (a) androcentricity (the world is viewed from the male perspective), (b) overgeneralization (a study dealing with one gender purports to apply to both), (c) sex insensitivity (gender is ignored as a socially and medically significant variable), and (d) double standards (identical behavior traits or situations are dealt with by different criteria).

Romm (1991) pointed out that, in the United States, "recent federal regulations require that women and minorities be adequately represented as subjects in appropriate research studies. Proposed research that does not include these groups will have to include an explanation for reviewers to assess whether the exclusion is justified" (p. 385).

A Checklist

It can be useful to consider a number of specific questions about the ethics of primary care research when considering a research project. As primary care providers, we may refer to people in our practices collectively as either patients or clients (an issue that warrants a separate discussion); in research, are they considered to be patients, clients, collaborators, partners, subjects, or volunteers? Will the same professional who provides service be conducting the research? What conflicts of values may arise? Will these conflicts be settled in favor of the net potential benefit accruing? How does one measure the quality of research, and against what criteria? Is the quality sufficient to warrant the risk and inconvenience to the patient and the expenditure of financial and personal resources on the part of the investigator? Are the measuring instruments appropriate, and, if technology dependent, are they well standardized and well maintained (e.g., are the blood pressure cuffs in hypertension studies standardized)?

Table 3.1 presents a checklist of questions that a primary care researcher might review in trying to account for all possible things.

Proposal or Grant Preparation

Nearly every granting agency has its own ethical guidelines, and these should be requested by researchers planning to develop a proposal. In general, it is safe to assume that no less than the Helsinki Declaration guidelines are acceptable. In an article on grantsmanship, Romm (1991) stated, "A statement of the applicants' understanding of potential harm as well as benefits will help reviewers understand the commitment to protecting the rights of study participants" (p. 385). All potential researchers would do well to write such a statement for each proposed study, regardless of their intent to seek funding for it.

Table 3.1 Checklist to Review Ethics of Research in Primary Care

A. Research Quality
   1. Is the research question worthy?
   2. Are the population, research design, measures, and sample size appropriate?

B. Consent
   1. Is consent to be given freely?
   2. Is consent to be given with full understanding? Are subjects competent to give consent?
   3. Are particularly vulnerable subjects given appropriate attention?

C. Confidentiality
   1. Are all data securely recorded and stored?
   2. Are subjects aware of how their information will be managed outside of their usual "for care" purposes?
   3. Will final reports be published in a manner ensuring confidentiality? If not, do the subjects consent?

D. Intervention
   1. Has a careful review of potential risks and benefits been completed?
   2. Is the researcher-provider in a true state of equipoise where an alternative to the "treatment" under study is employed as a "control" (be it no treatment, placebo, or a currently accepted treatment)?
   3. Is there a plan to stop the study according to an external, objective determination of benefit and harm (or risk of harm)?
   4. Is the client-professional (e.g., patient-doctor) relationship under continuous review for determination of harm?
   5. Can subjects withdraw from the study without fear of impairing their ongoing care?

E. Funding
   1. Can the source and nature of funding be shown not to affect the design, methodology, results, analysis, or publication of the study?

F. Collaboration
   1. Is there a clear understanding among research team members about distribution of responsibilities and credit?

Funding

A major decision to be made by the ethical clinician-researcher is whether financial support of research should be accepted from sponsors who have the potential to gain from a particular outcome of that research. If the funder can influence the study's design, implementation, analysis, or publication in any way that affects the outcome, the financial support should be rejected.

More subtle is the determination of the research question's origin: Is the study sponsor-driven or investigator-driven? Certain research groups accept a need to conduct studies of primary interest to industry in order to establish a funding base to conduct other studies of greater interest to themselves as investigators but that are not otherwise successfully funded. Some would argue that in a real, private enterprise world, this approval is acceptable as long as all of the studies involved answer worthy questions and are conducted in an ethical manner. Others would argue that any investigator who pursues questions that are not of primary personal interest in order to earn money for other research is expending energy and expertise inappropriately. Most health professional organizations include directions for these situations within their ethical guidelines, including the Canadian Nurses Association (1983), the British Psychological Society (1977), and the American Anthropological Association (Spradley, 1980). Private industry organizations that sponsor research (e.g., PMAC, 1990) and public agencies (e.g., the Medical Research Council of Canada, 1987) publish guidelines as well.

A further funding concern is whether research subjects should profit beyond the recovery of their expenses (which may include recognition of lost time). Advocates for the poor argue that financial incentives used to recruit economically disadvantaged persons to participate in research are unacceptable; some research groups have produced guidelines that specifically address this concern.

Quality Assessment or Research?

Responsible health care professionals monitor their own and each other's performance. This monitoring requires reviews and measures of the process of care, as well as assessments of its outcomes (the basic elements of much research). Public institutions are increasingly demanding ongoing accountability of individual practitioners' competence.

Where does quality assessment end and research begin? It is difficult to determine a difference between the two on the basis of the need to apply ethical standards. However, if the initial premise is accepted that primary care, primary care research, and the ethics of both are inextricably bound together in the personal relationship between provider and recipient, then there may be no need for such a differentiation.

One could argue that an ethical practitioner, by definition, is one who maintains a high standard of competence that can only be achieved and assessed by ongoing assessment of process and outcomes of care. Do clients/patients need to give consent for review of their records as part of ongoing quality assessment? I would argue that such self-assessment of professional perform-ance in the context of an individual practitioner's practice popu-lation is integral to its quality and is a reasonable expectation of any person seeking care from that practitioner. The assumption is that the standards of care applied are of a level expected by a reasonable, current, and prudent practitioner of similar kind. It is when a new management strategy or technique, insufficiently proven by generally accepted criteria, is to be introduced on trial, or when data collected from clients of that practice population are to be pooled with others or shared with others who are not part of the individual practitioner's care team, that the situation deserves "research" status and requires formal ethical standards of research to be applied.

What should be done if a potential client/patient chooses not to have personal information manipulated in any way, for pur-poses of quality assessment or otherwise, and without prejudice in terms of access and provision of care? In this situation, those who would argue for the practitioner's rights would allow that the practitioner, in keeping with an interest in providing care of acceptable quality, may choose not to accept that individual as a client. In my view, however, it is not appropriate at all for a practi-tioner not to accept or to dismiss a client for declining to partici-pate in research.

Advocacy for One's Patients Involved in Another's Study

Primary care providers refer patients to other professionals for consultation, for participation in assessment and management, and even for transferral of care. Many consultants are researchers as well, conducting studies on their own or taking part in large-scale, multicenter trials. Studies have been reported in which patients referred to consultants suffered harm in being assigned to no-treatment groups without knowledge of their randomized, no-treatment status (Paul, 1988) or in which the quality of the information given to them was insufficient for their making an informed choice to participate or not (Lynoe, Sandlund, Dahlgvist, & Jacobson, 1991). The primary care clinician, having a continuing concern for the patient, is responsible for being aware of the research activities of such consultants and having a clear working understanding with them about approaching and involving referred patients in such studies.

Computers

With the establishment of computers and other kinds of information technology, confidentiality becomes even more of a concern than it is with paper records. When certain aspects of information are transmitted outside of the service unit of care, such as happens with third-party payers for billing purposes, special concern must be applied to its control and management. Similarly, for research purposes, where data network joining is so easily possible with today's technology, special attention is necessary. At our university, for example, where we are about to bring together a data base from four primary care medical facilities serving more than 20,000 patients, we have established a specific committee to deal with data security. The relevant literature base is growing rapidly, and significant government legislation is being developed—for example, in Ontario, on the "Principles for Proposed Legislation on Health Care Information, Access and Privacy" (Freedom of Information and Protection of Privacy Act, 1990).

Conclusion

It is easy to be discouraged from doing research when one reviews the many ethical considerations presented here. However, every service-related encounter with people who seek health care involves the application of ethics. In primary care, where the interpersonal interaction is so basic to the process, the manner in which research ought to be conducted—that is, how ethically—can be guided by principles similar to those applied in providing service. Doing good, avoiding harm, encouraging autonomy, and striving for social justice are basic to both service and research endeavors, and primary health care professionals should be no strangers to these principles in their service activities. To extend them into research is but one further step; mostly it requires thoughtful consideration and consultation with those who have gone before.

References

Ashworth, C. (1981). Informed consent: When is it needed? *Family Medicine, 13,* 21.

Beauchamp, T. L., & Childress, J. F. (1979). *The Nuremberg Code in principles of biomedical ethics.* New York: Oxford University Press.

British Psychological Society. (1977). Ethics of investigations with human subjects: A set of principles proposed by the Scientific Affairs Board. *Bulletin of the British Psychological Society, 30,* 25-26.

Canadian Nurses Association. (1983). *Ethical guidelines for nursing involving human subjects.* Ottawa: Author.

Cassell, E. J. (1976). *The healer's art.* Philadelphia: J. B. Lippincott.

Cohen, M. (1991). Gender issues in family medicine research. *Canadian Family Physician, 37,* 1399-1405.

Coulehan, J. L., Shaffner, K. D., & Block, M. (1985). Ethics of clinical trials in family medicine. *Journal of Family Practice, 21,* 217-222.

Eimerl, T. S., & Laidlaw, A. J. (1969). *A handbook for research in general practice.* London: E & S Livingstone.

Frankel, M. S. (1972, February). The public service guidelines involving human subjects: An analysis of the policy making process [Monograph #10]. *Program of Policy Studies in Science and Technology.* Washington, DC: George Washington University.

Freedman, B. (1987). Equipoise and the ethics of clinical research. *New England Journal of Medicine, 317,* 141-145.

Freedom of Information and Protection of Privacy Act R.S.O. (1990). C.F. 31.

Glaser, E. M. (1964). Volunteers, controls, placebos, and questionnaires. In L. J. Witts (Ed.), *Medical surveys and clinical trials II* (p. 116). New York: Oxford University Press.

Hellman, S., & Hellman, D. (1991). Of mice but not men: Problems of the randomized clinical trial. *New England Journal of Medicine, 324,* 1585-1589.

Howie, J. G. R. (1979). *Research in general practice.* London: Croom Helm.

Lewis, J., MacLachlan, R. A., Labrecque, M., Herbert, C. P., Grava-Gubins, I., & Nickle, J. (1988). *The working group on the national recording system.* Mississauga, Ontario: College of Family Physicians of Canada.

Lynch, A. (1990, August). Placebo controlled trials in terminally ill patients: What place compassion? *Nova Scotia Medical Journal,* pp. 118-121.

Lynoe, N., Sandlund, M., Dahlgvist, G., & Jacobson, L. (1991). Informed consent: Study of quality of information given to participants in a clinical trial. *British Medical Journal, 303,* 610-613.

Mackenzie, J. (1917). *Principles of diagnosis and treatment in heart affections.* London: Oxford University Press.

Medical Research Council of Canada. (1987). *Guidelines on research involving human subjects.* Ottawa: Minister of Supplies and Services.

Meslin, E., & Lowy, F. H. (1990, March). *Research involving human subjects: "How" and "why" be ethical? Part 3.* Presented at a lecture series sponsored by the University of Toronto Centre for Biomedical Ethics, Toronto.

Pasamani, E. (1991). Clinical trials—Are they ethical? *New England Journal of Medicine, 324,* 1589-1591.

Paul, C. (1988). The New Zealand cervical cancer study: Could it happen again? *British Medical Journal, 297,* 533-539.

Pickles, W. (1939). *Epidemiology in country practice.* Baltimore: Williams & Wilkins.

PMAC Code of Marketing Practices. (1990). Ottawa: Pharmaceutical Manufacturers Association of Canada.

Public Health Service. (1969, May). *U.S. Department of Health, Education, and Welfare: Protection of the individual as a research subject.* Washington, DC: Author.

Revised Regulations of Ontario. (1970). O. Reg. 729, *48,* 5-6.

Romm, F. J. (1991). Practical grantsmanship: The application process in health care research. *Family Medicine, 23,* 382-386.

Shaffer, H. B. (1972). Medical ethics. In *Editorial research reports on medical issues* (p. 4). Washington, DC: Congressional Quarterly.

Spradley, J. P. (1980). *Participant observation.* New York: Holt, Rinehart & Winston.

Veatch, R. (1990). Should we study the Hippocratic oath? *Journal of Clinical Ethics, 1,* 292.

Watson, G. I. (1982). *Epidemiology and research in general practice.* London: Devonshire.

Weston, W., Brown, J. B., & Stewart, M. A. (1989). Patient-centred interviewing. Part I: Understanding patients' experiences. *Canadian Family Physician, 35,* 147-151.

PART II

Practical Issues

The practitioner who has a research idea that he or she thinks is worth pursuing may be able to forge ahead but likely will stumble on one of the many traps that await the unwary. In the following five chapters, experienced family practice researchers share their experience and expertise and point out many of the pitfalls.

Dr. Levenstein chronicles his development as a researcher while conducting a busy practice. He stresses the clinical origins of his research questions, the need to smoothly integrate research activity and clinical care and to involve the office staff.

Dr. Farley reviews the variety of factors that lead to patient involvement in research, paramount being the doctor-patient relationship. He identifies areas of practice organization that facilitate patient enrollment and retention in research.

Dr. Borkan introduces the developing area of qualitative research in the practice setting. He shows how qualitative methods are particularly useful for answering questions about patient behavior. He outlines the strengths, weaknesses, and uses of the three common methods: participant observation, long interviews, and focus groups.

Drs. Hogg and Lemelin illustrate the research potential of the office computer through examples from their rural practice. They offer suggestions for collecting clinical data that will be useful for research, and they consider the cost implications.

Drs. Morris and Almagor illustrate the value of looking beyond the office to the surrounding community. From his Canadian setting, Morris presents examples of research responding to community needs. Almagor presents an Israeli example of a practice developed to be community oriented.

These five chapters deal only with some of the myriad of practical issues of practice research. For additional items I refer the reader to the appendix, "Checklist for Conducting Research in the Practice Setting," which summarizes the issues identified by the authors and adds others.

4 Combining Clinical Care and Research

JOSEPH H. LEVENSTEIN

For the family physician or primary care provider interested in combining research and clinical care, selecting the topic to research is a reflection of one's personality and interests, rather than of the need to meet a prescribed research agenda. There is a temptation, when discussing this subject, to chronicle all of the major contributors and their approaches; however, I thought it would be more illustrative to share my own biases, interests, thought processes, doubts, limitations, and, most important, my own personal development as a family physician. This development has evolved during more than 20 years of doing both patient care and research.

I will not here refer to any of the studies in which I was involved that took place in academic settings, but only those that emanated from our three-person university-affiliated family practice, where we each saw, on average, 20 to 30 patients per day. In any of these studies that involved collaboration, the other participants also were active community practitioners, seeing a similar number of patients.

One of the major impediments I find when discussing research with young family physicians is the difficulty in changing the traditional medical research mind-set of those searching for a research proposal. It is one I can empathize with, particularly as I am a product of the early phases of family medicine's evolution to a discipline in the late 1960s and early 1970s. (We came from a world that purported to give certainty into a world that gave anything but.)

Qualities of a Researcher

One cannot overstate the fact that the essential characteristics needed in a researcher are more attitudinal than purely academic. There must be an interest at least, a passion at best, in order to answer a question or to validate a theory. Perhaps none has put it better than Howie (1991) what constitutes a good research question: It must be of interest, answerable, and ultimately of importance. Also needed is the discipline to do the literature review, design and execute the protocols, assemble the results, and prepare the article, and the willingness to obtain help where necessary. So research, to me, is the challenging question and the self-discipline to carry the inquiry through. As part of the earlier vanguard of the discipline, there was also a desire to establish our scientific foundations and legitimacy.

Study on Prehospital Management of Acute Myocardial Infarction

So much by way of introduction; now for my journey. I entered general practice with no formal training in the discipline but with a strong tradition and value system of the vocation having been inculcated in me. (Many of my family were doctors, most general practitioners.) I knew the value and importance of caring even if I did not fully understand the implications.

In fact, I was not even sure I was going to remain in general practice; I was passionately interested in cardiology, particularly the management of acute myocardial infarction in the intensive coronary care unit (ICCU) (Levenstein, 1976b). Lives were being saved by reversing or preventing arrhythmias in "hearts too good to die." An extensive review of the literature, however, showed that the hospital, despite halving the death rate in the ICCU, was having a negligible impact on the community death rate: Most victims were dying *prior* to hospitalization, from preventable and reversible arrhythmias, within hours of the onset of symptoms (Levenstein, 1971). It appeared that to reduce the death rate significantly, the community, not the hospital, was the place to do it. I rationalize that this observation was the turning point in my commitment to remain in general practice, but I was probably hooked anyway.

Hospital-based medicine was not slow to hone in on this area and began to extend itself into the community with mobile intensive coronary care units (MICCUs), paramedics, and sophisticated technology. All of this equipment and personnel, however, was at great cost and with tremendous administrative problems. What if we in general practice could show that the general practitioner who serves a circumscribed area and has knowledge of his or her patients at risk, having been educated with a simple protocol, the main objectives of which were a prompt response, treatment, and prevention of the premonitory arrhythmias and the alleviation of pain, could, in the management of prehospital acute myocardial infarction, effect a service that compared with that of a MICCU (Levenstein, 1976a, 1982a)?

At the time, I thought my proposal was pure biomedicine as applied to general practice. Looking at it today, I see that it was loaded with the unique characteristics of our discipline. The research group debated the merits of a control group, but as we were, in effect, measuring a health care delivery approach with multiple variables, we finally opted for a carefully monitored collaborative case study with more than 100 GPs participating (Levenstein, 1976a). The year-long study involved endless organization, administration with contact persons in every hospital, liaison with every cardiologist in town, and even contact with the morgue, lest a sudden death somehow went unreported.

One concept I learned early on and that I applied to this study was that once some organization is in place, you are able to look at peripheral questions for not too much extra trouble. We were able to address not only the central question but others also, including the natural history of acute heart attacks (Levenstein, 1982c), the identification of the circumstances prior to heart attack, and the value of research as a means of continuing medical education (Levenstein, 1976c).

EARLY LESSONS

Do not misunderstand me: I do not suggest for one moment that multipractice research is the way for anyone to start out. What this example does illustrate, however, is that if the question is burning enough, one can move mountains—with some help—to effect a project.

Furthermore the question was a burning one to my collaborators as well. Do not try to persuade collaborators to join if they are not interested; it will backfire almost without exception and is far more trouble than it is worth. Reluctant collaborators were less prepared to make additional commitments or to attend meetings involving education, modification of the protocols, and ultimate agreement in all aspects of the study. Eventually, in collaborative studies, we developed a system whereby we wrote to potential investigators, informing them of an upcoming study and asking them to reply in writing. If they accepted, they then had to attend an investigators' meeting. This simple approach ensured a low dropout rate by weeding out less enthusiastic participants at the start. A method that failed us was inviting doctors whom we knew to be sympathetic to participate. Invariably they all agreed, but more, I believe, to accommodate our request than because they were interested or committed.

Another notable lesson learned from this and other endeavors was that the research project had to be almost an integral part of the GP's job definition and not involve untold additional activities. It is useless doing an anticoagulant study or a natural history study on the early changes of full routine neurological examinations if neither activity is part of the GP's usual job definition. While accepting that a study inevitably must involve performing some activities outside normal patient care, it is essential that these be limited; otherwise, interest must wane due to the day-to-day realities of treating a full patient load. Also there must be some direct benefit to patient care. For example, in the acute myocardial infarction study, all of the GPs did house calls and also had, from 1 to 8 times a year, depending on the age spread of the practice, patients with suspected heart attacks. Suspected heart attacks were most often referred to the hospital emergency department. The study mandated a house call *immediately* if an acute myocardial infarction was suspected—a slight but acceptable modification of practice. Finally the design of the study recording form allowed it to serve as the data base for the study and as both a referral note and a record for the doctor.

The issue of time has to be addressed, as well, because we are dealing with practitioners whose primary purpose is to care for patients. Although lack of time may often be used as a rationalization not to do research, it does represent a real problem for the busy clinician. All components of research take time, with the amount dependent on the role played by the investigator. A principal investigator who is designing protocols and executing literature reviews obviously has to have designated hours for this activity or else use leisure time. The key problem regarding time, however, relates to the activities that take place during actual patient care. Ideally the time spent on research here must be limited and the activities related as far as possible to legitimate patient care behavior.

Another extremely important lesson was the value of the carefully documented prospective case study as a contribution to knowledge. In fact, the bulk of medicine is made up from meticulously recorded observations. I vividly recall being challenged and never believed regarding my results at cardiology conferences. "Where were your controls?" was the question frequently asked. However, these surgeons and physicians rarely had any controls themselves, having themselves introduced a plethora of technological interventions and diagnostic modalities yet to be rigorously evaluated. So yet another lesson is that you have to believe in simple, careful description and not feel that every study has to have a blinded, randomized design.

We were able to conclude, among other things, that in the prehospital phase of acute myocardial infarction, the study physicians were able to administer a service that compared favorably with an MICCU, at almost no extra cost to the community and with very little strain on their practices (Levenstein, 1976a, 1982a). At the time, this research had very little impact in North America, but in the present economic times it may well warrant a second look.

QUESTIONS ARISING FROM THE STUDY

Many other questions arose out of the acute myocardial infarction study that led to my conducting observational natural history case and intervention studies on angina (Levenstein, 1978c, 1980), hypertension (Levenstein, 1978a), and complete home management of myocardial infarction (Levenstein, 1982b). One of the study outcomes that troubled me was that although the sudden death rate had been reduced dramatically by addressing one of the variables that is so important to our discipline—a well-educated, promptly responding doctor—I had overlooked another: the patient variable. Most of the delays now were caused by patients, and it was often a delay of days rather than hours. Our survey into the patients who experienced a sudden death showed a definite profile: They were hypertensive and/or had angina and/or had premonitory cardiac symptoms that, at least in retrospect, should have led to alarm bells ringing (Levenstein, 1982c). However, they had elected not to seek medical help. If we as general practitioners are continuously managing patients long before catastrophic events, surely we can isolate those at risk and manage their defense mechanisms, as well as their risk factors and manifest disease, long before they literally drop dead. As a result of these observations, I undertook studies in my practice that led to two papers on the emergency management of preinfarction angina in general practice and the predictability of acute heart attacks (Levenstein, 1978c, 1982a). Both were predominantly observational natural history case studies, the very basis of medicine. I belabor this point because many family medicine researchers miss important opportunities for within-practice research by undervaluing this approach. These studies will provide the basis for further testing of results and hypotheses in controlled designs.

Lest the point has gone unnoticed, my ventures into research had the effect of totally immersing me in the *principles* of family medicine. I have found the most crucial of these to be that although biomedical premises rarely introduce the doctor, the patient, and their relationship as variables, these are fundamental to the thinking of family medicine (Levenstein, 1988, 1990).

A Research Project Addressing
Family Physician Practice Dilemmas

To continue with the theme of solving burning issues in any subject that affects family medicine/general practice, the doctors in our area were involved in an after-hours call system. This process evoked annoyance among certain participants, who felt they were doing more visits than others on their nights on duty.

We set up a study on doctor and patient attitudes to after-hours calls (Levenstein, 1981a) in order to assess what really was happening. The study had several phases. First, we would agree among ourselves and then document what constitutes "reasonable grounds" to execute an after-hours visit. We then would monitor all of our phone calls after hours and record the problem and our action— that is, "advice"; "visit," which meant seeing patients mainly at home or at the office; or meeting them at the hospital. A third piece of information was a survey that obtained patients' attitudes to these after-hours calls—for example, for what reason did they call, what were their expectations, what responses did they expect? Several questions were based on the patients' perceived behavior by the doctors. Finally we would meet to compare and log our charts and to discuss our phone call rate/visit rate and how this ratio related to our agreed-upon criteria and the patients' expectations.

The doctors were more or less divided into two groups: those with a high visit-to-phone-call ratio and those with a low ratio. Analysis for the documented "reasons for a doctor visit" could not explain this difference. The rationalizations prior to the study were once again offered—namely, that visits were "expected," "insisted upon," or "wanted" by the patient. However, these items did not square with our patient survey results. The doctors had to look to their own behavior, and it became evident that it was their responses and behavior more than the patients' that was prompting unnecessary after-hours visits. To quote one physician's remark: "My anger at doing an 'unnecessary' visit is overridden by my anxiety at missing something."

After the study discussions, doctors reported that they were able to cope far better with "unnecessary" calls, and their phone call/visit rates dropped accordingly.

The Value of Preregistration Drug Studies to Family Medicine Research

There are several compelling reasons to do third-phase preregistration drug trials: (a) Only 10% of such trials are executed in the community, yet 90% of medicines are prescribed in the community, (b) they are extremely well remunerated, and most important of all, (c) the organizational infrastructure allows one to look at other questions as well as the actual medicine trial itself.

I was principal investigator in a number of very important third-phase preregistration drug trials. I will not discuss these per se, as this issue is covered in Chapter 11; however, I want to allude briefly to a research spin-off that developed.

In a double-blind controlled study on the first-ever beta blocker and diuretic combination versus methyldopa, the side effects at various stages of the study were monitored (Levenstein, 1978b, 1981b). Far more side effects were elicited from the patients in the placebo run-in period than throughout the study either on the treatment or control medicine. One could only assume that the patients got tired of mentioning symptoms that may often be present under normal circumstances. Thereafter, in all future studies, we had a compelling argument to claim that the best way to question patients about relevant side effects would be simply to ask them "how they felt on the medicine." Several pharmaceutical companies now have adopted this approach.

Another spin-off of a drug trial was that natural history data are produced that are useful to the practitioner. In a double-blind controlled study to assess a new antibiotic in the treatment of bacteriologically significant urinary tract infection (UTI), the protocol was amended so that patients were entered prior to the culture result and could be continued in the study even if the count grew less than 100,000 organisms/ml (Levenstein, 1986). The additional purposes of this study were to see whether there were any predictors to a bacteriologically significant UTI in the community, to examine the criteria by which GPs clinically adjudged a UTI to be potentially bacteriologically significant, and to note whether doctors changed their behavior after receiving the results of a nonsignificant bacteriuria. The treatment was 10 days both on the trial drug and the control drug, and the culture result was received within 24 to 48 hours (Levenstein, 1993).

The results were fascinating. First, no discriminatory factors on urine examination were found to indicate specifically the bacteriological outcome. For example, the number of pus cells in the urine did not help, being poorly sensitive and specific for a UTI. Furthermore the criteria for treatment were patient symptoms and signs and *anything* abnormal in the urine. Finally, once the doctors had made their diagnoses, they ignored the culture result. In short, they ignored the conventional criteria for a 10-day treatment of a UTI, rather favoring to manage the clinical symptoms. What was, at face value, a randomized trial of an antibiotic also provided excellent insights into issues important to office practice.

Finally, I would like to report the findings of a multicentered trial on a new prophylactic medicine versus placebo for asthma (Levenstein, 1991). Nearly 2,000 patients were entered from 14 countries, and every parameter was measured, including three functional status surveys: patient diary cards, days of work illness incidents, and lung function tests.

The new drug did lead to an improvement in asthma patients in certain parameters; however, the addition of all of the extra measures for patient care and for recording of data, including more doctor visits, patient diary cards, and regular phone calls, gave us insight into how many parameters improved and by how much in the placebo group. Attention alone improved patients' status in several physical, psychological, social, and functional status parameters.

A crucial point in relation to examining additional questions in drug studies, or any other type of study for that matter, is that these must be defined prospectively and the protocols added to accordingly.

Early Detection of Disease

Another example of where we set about doing a collaborative study was occult blood screening for detection of carcinoma of the colon, involving more than 3,000 patients and more than 100 doctors (Elliot, Levenstein, & Wright, 1984a, 1984b; Levenstein & Elliot, 1982). This study differed from others in the literature in that the blood testing was to be done in two phases and that GPs would distribute the tests, which would be centrally evaluated, with patients returning them in the mail. The hope was that these processes would increase patient adherence, compared to other studies in which only one test was mailed to the patient for mail return and included dietary and other restrictions. In our study the first phase involved testing without any restrictions on meat or medications, for example. Only if the occult blood was positive was the patient then retested with restrictions.

Similar to other studies, only 1% of the patients subsequently were found to have had malignant or premalignant conditions. What we did not expect was that the "compliance" rate was only as good as the upper figures of other studies: 70%. We had expected a higher rate and hypothesized that this might have been the case had the GPs been involved during the whole process, with the tests being returned to them rather than to a central point.

Clinical Process of Family Medicine

An area that has always fascinated me is the clinical process of family medicine where one is dealing largely with undifferentiated illness. I was spurred into action by a medical student who had been with me for an entire day and demanded to know how I could deal with this vast array of problems in such a relatively short time. I then set out to audiotape and later to videotape 1,000 of my interactions to observe what I was doing intuitively (Levenstein, 1984). My clinical process proved to be definable by an extremely simple schema, and it formed the basis of the patient-centered method that we refined and researched at The University of Western Ontario (Brown, Stewart, McCracken, McWhinney, & Levenstein, 1986; Levenstein, McCracken, McWhinney, Stewart, & Brown, 1986; Stewart, Brown, Levenstein, McCracken, & McWhinney, 1986).

Research Process in Retrospect

Central throughout my research activity was a burning desire to answer a question or to learn something. The process then became to refine the question into an answerable form or hypothesis that was congruent with carrying out my general practice. The decision to perform it singly or collaboratively depended on finances and/or on whether other colleagues might be interested. I was also more likely to go it alone if the hypothesis was based on a personal observation or was related specifically to my practice. Then came the organization and the consultation with colleagues in and out of the discipline to define the protocol.

Help is not only necessary but crucial, as one often overlooks glaring deficiencies. Finally came the execution of the studies.

In truth, I became more interested in the variables that are not taken into account in traditional biomedicine—namely, the doctor, the patient, and what goes on between them—only later to learn, to my eternal joy, that this relativism is pure new Einstein/ Heisenberg physics (Levenstein, 1988, 1990). I also appeared, in clinical practice research, to have favored the natural historian method (which I can truthfully aver was more by accident than by any conscious design). I also was able to write theoretical papers on the principles and science of family medicine, largely, I think, because of my intense involvement in actual practice and research.

Additional Issues

A number of additional issues related to research in clinical practice must be addressed. Patient participation and cooperation are essential. The benefits to patients and to medicine in general must be explained carefully, in addition to obtaining informed consent. This procedure gets easier as the process continues. After a number of years, patients would start to ask me, "Any new study we can participate in?" Also, if there is benefit to the patient from a new medicine, it is essential to negotiate continuation of this medicine after the study period has ended. We, more than anyone else, should not "use" patients.

A related point is that we must be aware that a research protocol, even when looking for qualitative data, alters our clinical process. The topic or clinical event under research can become all-embracing, and we can become very doctor centered. I remember one specific incident in which a patient wanted to talk about her back problems, but as it had been a doctor-initiated visit to see whether she would fit into an asthma study, I had not taken her needs into account at all. This attitude can be counterproductive to acceptable patient care, with patient problems being missed or ignored.

The involvement of office staff is crucial: They must be aware of and buy into the study. Inevitably it involves additional work and commitment on their part, so in some instances appropriate remuneration should be offered. Even more important, determined efforts should be made to include them in attendance at investigator meetings; to explain protocols, objectives, and the knowledge and benefit to patient care that can be derived; to include them on the newsletter mailing list; and to keep them up to date on the study's progress.

Although clinical research on family medicine questions never seems to attract much money, assistance is often essential. In collaborative studies, with their technical and administrative needs, a research assistant or monitor is obligatory. Collecting and checking forms, contacting patients, collating laboratory results, and arranging meetings are activities beyond the capabilities of a busy practicing clinician. Grant money usually can be obtained for this activity from academies or colleges of family medicine, for example; and, of course, when an additional study is being piggybacked onto a drug study, that infrastructure is already in place. Smaller groups of perhaps 8 to 10 doctors, geographically closely situated, sometimes can get by with the budget of a drug representative who uses the opportunity to be able to simultaneously contact the doctor directly and do the administration.

Individual studies often require very little technology. I used a method of notebooks that I learned from John Fry for certain topics or conditions, with pages for each patient whose folder had previously been identified. Computers were used initially only to analyze data, and only later as an adjunct to patient population definition and tracing. At the risk of being labeled a heretic, the lack of practice computer facilities should not be used as a rationalization not to participate in research. Needless to say, however, they are a boon to those who use them. Assistance for researchers in practice is usually available in the local academy/college or a nearby department of family medicine, and practitioners should make every effort to contact these resources.

Ultimately clinical research in the community is where our discipline is most likely to be defined because our academic departments of family medicine are "artificial" to some extent by virtue of the patient population, lack of continuing care, or the importance of other priorities such as teaching.

GPs can participate in research in many ways, and some doctors are better in one or another area of activity. They can be principal investigators, collaborators, additional observers or participants, administrators, reviewers, technical advisors to protocols, methodologists, or analyzers of results. Everyone need not do everything. The key problem I have always found is to instill in GPs the belief that they *can* do research and that family medicine *is* a valid arena for research.

Finally I need hardly remind readers that every interaction with a patient is an "experiment"—not only an experiment, but a human experience that we can influence by our knowledge, attitudes, and skills, bearing in mind that the outcome will be profoundly affected by the patient as well. Within this framework, the research possibilities are limitless. We have an imperative, however, to focus on those activities that are peculiar to our situation.

References

Brown, J., Stewart, M. A., McCracken, E., McWhinney, I. R., & Levenstein, J. H. (1986). The patient-centered clinical method 2: Definition and application. *Family Practice—An International Journal, 3*(2), 75-79.

Elliot, M. E., Levenstein, J. H., & Wright, P. R. (1984a). The early detection of colonic cancer by haemoccult screening test. *British Journal of Surgery, 7*, 785-788.

Elliot, M. E., Levenstein, J. H., & Wright, P. R. (1984b). The results of the Cape general practice haemoccult screening survey. *South African Medical Journal, 66*, 219-221.

Howie, J. G. R. (1991). Refining questions and hypotheses. In P. G. Norton, M. Stewart, F. Tudiver, M. J. Bass, & E. V. Dunn (Eds.), *Primary care research: Traditional and innovative approaches* (pp. 13-25). Newbury Park, CA: Sage.

Levenstein, J. H. (1971). The role of the general practitioner in the early management of acute myocardial infarction. *South African Medical Journal, 45*, 1103-1109.

Levenstein, J. H. (1976a). Emergency management of acute myocardial infarction by the general practitioner. *South African Medical Journal, 50*, 531-538.

Levenstein, J. H. (1976b). Myocardial infarction and the evolution of the intensive coronary care unit. *South African Medical Journal, 50*, 918-926.

Levenstein, J. H. (1976c). A research project as a means of continuing education. *Journal of the Royal College of General Practitioners, 26*, 384-386.

Levenstein, J. H. (1978a). Observations of hypertension in general practice. *Elan Journal of Faculty of General Practice, 34*, 9-13.

Levenstein, J. H. (1978b). Oxprenolol slow release with cyclopenthiazide KCl compared with methyldopa in the treatment of essential hypertension. *South African Medical Journal, 54*(Part 1), 860-869.

Levenstein, J. H. (1978c). The treatment of the emergency crescendo (reinfarction) angina. *Elan Journal of Faculty of General Practice, 24*, 7-12.

Levenstein, J. H. (1980). The emergency treatment of crescendo angina. *Journal of the Royal College of General Practitioners*, Occasional Paper 10. Selected articles from the 8th World Conference of Family Physicians.

Levenstein, J. H. (1981a). After-hours visits—Doctors' and patients' attitudes. *South African Medical Journal, 60*(1), 19-23.

Levenstein, J. H. (1981b). Oxprenolol slow release with cyclopenthiazide KCl in the treatment of essential hypertension. *South African Medical Journal, 59*(Part II), 900-904.

Levenstein, J. H. (1982a, March). A comparison between delivery care systems in the early pre-hospital phase of acute myocardial infarction. *Update*, pp. 846-854.

Levenstein, J. H. (1982b, May). Home versus hospital care of myocardial infarction. *Update*, pp. 1785-1791.

Levenstein, J. H. (1982c). The natural history of acute heart attacks: Cape GP survey. *South African Medical Journal, 6*, 863-866.

Levenstein, J. H. (1984). The patient-centered general practice consultation. *South African Journal of Family Practice, 7*, 276-282.

Levenstein, J. H. (1986). Comparison of cefixime and co-trimoxazole in acute uncomplicated urinary tract infection: A double-blind general practice study. *South African Medical Journal, 70*, 455-460.

Levenstein, J. H. (1988). Family medicine and the new science. *South African Journal of Family Practice, 9*(1), 11-17.

Levenstein, J. H. (1990). Symptom interpretation: The crux of clinical competence. *South African Journal of Family Practice, 11*, 54-59.

Levenstein, J. H. (1991). Quality of life, symptoms and pulmonary function in asthma: A year-long multi-center double-blind trial of nedocromil sodium versus placebo. *Family Practice, 8*(4), 402-403.

Levenstein, J. H. (1993). *Urinary tract infections in the community.* Unpublished manuscript.

Levenstein, J. H., & Elliot, M. E. (1982). Haemoccult screening for colorectal carcinoma in general practice. *South African Journal of Family Practice, 5*, 252-256.

Levenstein, J. H., McCracken, E., McWhinney, I. R., Stewart, M. A., & Brown, J. B. (1986). The patient-centered clinical method 1: A model for the doctor/patient interaction in family medicine. *Family Practice—An International Journal, 3*(1), 24-30.

Stewart, M. A., Brown, J. B., Levenstein, J. H., McCracken, E. C., & McWhinney, I. R. (1986). The patient-centered clinical method 3: Changes in residents' performance over two months of training. *Family Practice—An International Journal, 3*(3), 164-167.

5   Recruiting and Retaining Patients in Research

EUGENE FARLEY

The factors involved in recruiting and retaining patients in practice-based research have much in common with those that affect patient compliance with interventions that have proven value in maintaining or regaining health. Often, however, involvement in a research project offers no immediate advantage to the patients; therefore, their willingness to participate has different implications.

Physicians and other providers involved in practice-based research find that most patients are willing to become involved: Participation is usually at a rate of 85% to 90% or higher when patients are approached by their own physicians. This statistic is confirmed from my own experiences in practice in a Navajo community (McDermott, Deuschle, Adair, Fulmer, & Loughlin, 1960), in rural upstate New York and in university teaching family practices, from discussions with other clinicians involved in practice-based research, and through a cursory review of the literature in selected family practice journals. The range of patient enrollment was from 45% to 95% of those approached.

Many of the factors determining this willingness can be influenced by the physician or investigators and can be recognized or identified easily from practical experience. They include:

The type of study proposed
The risks, time, and inconvenience involved
The presence or absence of invasive procedures

The potential value to others

The quality of the provider/patient relationship, including commitment of the former to the study

The nature of the practice

The practice management

The number and types of personnel serving in the practice

The presence or absence of active patient education

The relationship of the practice to the community

The previous involvement of the practice in research projects

The role of learners (students and residents) in the practice

The characteristics of the population served

Whether or not subjects are paid for their time or inconvenience

The social or moral implications of the problem under study (such as HIV positivity and AIDS)

The confidence in the ability of the practice to maintain confidentiality if such is desired

The public awareness of and attitude toward the problem being studied

These factors are discussed in detail below.

TYPE OF STUDY, RISKS, TIME
AND INCONVENIENCE, PRESENCE
OR ABSENCE OF PROCEDURES,
AND POTENTIAL VALUE TO OTHERS

When a practice-based research project is being developed, serious consideration must be given to the type of study and to its impact on both the patients and providers. Any study in which patients are involved directly requires clear understanding by all participants of its purpose, procedures, risks, potential outcomes for the subject, and potential significance for others.

Most practice-based research requires minimal to moderate input from the patient, is associated with no risk, and requires only minor changes in the practice. Studies that have low risk and that offer the greatest potential good to society are the ones most readily accepted by patients. Clinical drug trials, especially in the prelicensure stage (Phase III), are the most demanding and disruptive of normal routine.

PROVIDER-PATIENT RELATIONSHIP

When permission is required, the provider-patient relationship can be a significant factor in patients' acceptance. If the practice is composed of a single provider and patients are able to choose other providers in the area, we can assume that they have selected that physician for various individual reasons and are satisfied with the doctor-patient relationship. In situations where patients have limited or no ability to select their personal providers, such as in isolated communities with one physician, in group practices, or because of restrictions of a health insurance plan, they may be less inclined to participate. For example, in Wisconsin, where employers must offer at least two health care programs, patients often are forced to change doctors when the employer changes insurers or program options on the basis of competitive costs. To receive care outside of work-related health care plan coverage is more expensive than most individuals can afford. Therefore, even in our university family medicine teaching practices, we gain and lose patients who would like to stay but are forced to change because their physician is not covered by a health program offered by their employer. Dr. David Hahn told me that, of the 18.7% of the patients who declined to participate in an asthma study (Hahn, Dodge, & Golubjatnikov, 1991), the majority were new to him and to the practice. Those patients with whom he had an established relationship not only participated willingly but at times also ask when he will be starting another study. If doctor-patient communications are open, there is mutual respect, the patient feels comfortable accepting or declining participation, and the study is clearly defined and explained, the probability is high that most patients will become interested.

Acceptance is also higher if the practice is organized so that patients know their doctor and the doctor, as well as the other providers—nurse practitioners, physician assistants, medical technicians, and receptionists—knows the patients, that is, if there is a sense of personal connection.

NATURE OF THE PRACTICE

Practice type, function, and structure are important determinants of what types of research can be done and of patient acceptance.

Traditionally, large, impersonal hospital clinics have had more difficulty with compliance than smaller, more personal private practices, yet often have been the predominant site for research on ambulatory populations. A study conducted specifically to compare the acceptance rate of patients from a small group family practice and an equivalent size academic practice showed a 3.3 times greater acceptance by the former (Wadland, Hughes, Secker-Walker, Bronson, & Fenwick, 1990). In my review of recent medical journals (mentioned earlier), however, little difference was found in the reported acceptance rate of studies conducted in these two types of environments. This finding seems contrary to common wisdom but may reflect the observation by individuals working in large public hospitals and in neighborhood clinics that patients develop great loyalty to any organization or institution from which they receive ongoing care. Despite differing enrollment rates, research needs to be done in all types of settings in which patients receive primary care.

The nature and size of a practice are also determinants of acceptance. Because of the type of problems seen, mixed-specialty practices may be able to undertake studies different from those of single-specialty practices, and primary care practices can undertake studies on a subset of the population different from those of subspecialty practices. For studies involving family members, family practices are more appropriate than specialty practices. Patients in a health maintenance organization (HMO) or prepaid practices may be more amenable to studies on prevention than patients in fee-for-service practices. Regardless of practice type, all depend on the commitment of their providers and on the loyalty, understanding, and interest of their patients.

PRACTICE MANAGEMENT

The way a practice is managed will affect patients' willingness to participate in research. Factors include how patients are scheduled with their physicians or other providers; how available the practitioners are to the patients; the hours the practice is open; how support staff relate to the providers, the patients, and the community; how the business office handles billings and collections (particularly for those who have difficulty paying or who receive Medicaid or Medicare benefits); and the general ambience of the facility.

How a practice organizes the data it collects in the ongoing care of patients helps determine the type of research that can be done. An important starting point is the minimal basic data set (MBDS) collected on all patients (see Chapter 7). Even if the MBDS includes only the usual registration data such as name, date of birth, address, telephone number, head of household, and insurance company or payor, there is an excellent basis on which to define research questions as well as to manage the practice if these data are retrievable so that the population served can be divided into cohorts. If the MBDS is expanded to include disease or problem, education, occupation, race, religion, ethnicity, and members of household, the variety of questions that can be asked and answered is increased dramatically. If these data are organized so that they can be retrieved easily, they are invaluable for identifying potential subjects for studies. Use of the morbidity index and age/sex register together allows the determination of such questions as how many of the individuals in the practice between the ages of 70 and 80 have been seen for the diagnosis of hypertension in the past 2 years, and who in the practice over 65 years and who below 65 years has a chronic lung or cardiac problem and therefore is in need of influenza immunization. Knowing how many single parents are in the practice and who they are facilitates the ability to study the specific problems of single parents. Practices with well-organized MBDS have an excellent opportunity to identify studies that need to be done, are relevant to the population served, and can be done with the active cooperation of the involved patients.

In an effort to determine the readiness of some teaching practices in the United States for practice-based research, I sent out a questionnaire to all 365 Family Practice Residency program directors in the United States to find out what parts of a minimal basic data set (MBDS) were already available across programs. Of the directors who answered (40%), representing 255 teaching practices, 72% have an active age/sex registry, 96% of which are computerized; and another 20% say they can get age/sex information with reasonable effort. Also 92% reported an ability to group their individual patients by provider, 85% by ZIP code, 73% by diagnosis or problem, 54% by head of household, 52% by family,

45% by race, 22% by census tract, 18% by ethnicity, 15% by occupation, 10% by religion, and 8.5% by education level.

PATIENT EDUCATION

Practices that place a high emphasis on patient education for health maintenance and disease prevention usually attract patients who are more motivated to remain in good health. Some of these practices use the services of a nurse practitioner or health educator, professionals who are usually very comfortable communicating with patients and often can be used to help recruit and retain them into studies. When such is the case, patient participation usually is excellent, particularly for studies that have some connection with health maintenance or disease prevention.

RELATIONSHIP TO THE COMMUNITY

Practices that use a community-oriented primary care (COPC) approach (Nutting, 1987) are involved fully in the community, have an advisory committee of community members, and work closely with the community to improve the overall health status of the population. One of the early COPC practices in the United States was the Navajo Cornell Clinic Practice in Arizona, serving a population living in an 800-square-mile area. Its success in patient care, outreach, and research was largely attributable to the very strong advisory committee, composed of representatives from the community, including medicine men. These individuals asked many questions that helped educate them, the providers, and the community. It gave the physicians, nurses, health visitors, and medical anthropologists an opportunity to work with the community on common health concerns; to explain what we could and could not do in the way of prevention, diagnosis, and treatment; and to explain what we were doing in the way of research. Committee members were involved with the clinic from its inception and had significant input throughout its existence. Their commitment enabled us to undertake studies on the prevalence and ambulatory treatment of TB, streptococcal disease, including rheumatic fever and glomerulonephritis, and on the general health of the population. Prevention, care, and research were truly a community affair. For the most part, COPC practices should have little problem enrolling and retaining patients in studies.

In the late 1960s and early 1970s, when the Rochester Neighbourhood Health Centers were being developed, the patients who were to be served by them specifically wanted to avoid the impersonalization they experienced in some of the hospital clinics and did not want to be "guinea pigs" for research or for the education of medical students or residents. This attitude rapidly changed once the members of the community board serving one of these health centers participated in the recruitment of family practice residents who would be working there through their 3 years of training. The whole atmosphere, sense of ownership, and community were different at the NHC than at the university hospital clinics. The developing sense of ownership, responsibility, and community pride that involved both the patients and the providers facilitated numerous practice studies by residents and others. When a community believes the practice group has a sense of responsibility toward its members, individuals are usually very willing to participate in research.

PREVIOUS INVOLVEMENT IN RESEARCH

If a practice or the providers within it have been involved in research in the past, and if patients there have had good experiences relative to the research, they usually will show a greater willingness to participate in other projects.

Practices that participate in research networks often inform patients of this through a placard in the waiting room (Beasley et al., 1991; Green et al., 1984). Most often, such participation is seen as evidence of dedication, which creates a sense of pride in both providers and patients.

ROLE OF LEARNERS

The role of learners, such as residents or medical, nursing, and physician assistant students, can have a significant impact. If these learners are integrated into the practice setting in a manner that wins patient acceptance and interest, they can increase the willingness of patients to participate in a specific project. If they are poorly integrated, patients may feel imposed on and may view research as just another infringement on their relationship with their physician or other provider.

From my own experience and that of others, practices that include medical students and other learners have no problem with patient involvement in research if the patients are made aware of the activities and feel included in the process and if the learners are monitored closely and have clearly delineated roles that are consistent with their learning stage.

NATURE OF POPULATION SERVED

Of basic importance in any practice-based research project is an understanding of the population served, as socioeconomic and sociocultural status may affect how an individual or group accepts involvement.

Some groups, because of clearly defined distinguishing attributes, make it easy for researchers to develop hypotheses or questions that practice- or population-based research may answer. In the diverse population of the United States are many subsets whose belief systems and/or life-styles are a major determinant of their members' health and illness. Cultural groups whose health or health behaviors have been studied in some detail include American Indians, Mormons, Seventh Day Adventists, Amish, and Hindus. Groups with culturally or religiously determined life-styles that differ from those of the general population provide us with natural experimental conditions, similar to those provided by geographic distances and differences, for comparing health outcomes. However, although such groups may present ideal opportunities for natural epidemiologic, population-based studies, some may have specific cultural beliefs or prohibitions that deter their members from participating (Clark, 1983).

With the diverse peoples who make up the North American continent and this world, it can be expected that practice-based research will come to focus increasingly on health and illness patterns associated with this diversity. We are finding this particularly true in some of our practices in Wisconsin, where we have had a large influx of new Americans from Southeast Asia, a growing influx of Hispanic and African Americans, and an increased awareness of American Indians. Many patients from these groups have beliefs about health and disease that differ markedly from those of the Euro-Americans, who have been the dominant group in Wisconsin for the past 150 years. In the Family Medicine Residency program of the University of Wisconsin, Mary Grow, our medical anthropologist, has developed an outreach program to the Southeast Asian and other minority populations we serve. The purpose of this outreach is to improve that population's understanding of prevention and what Western medicine has to offer them, and to help our physicians understand their health belief systems so that we can better serve them. Already this outreach has led to some practice-based research on health care issues important to this population, including one on fundal height during pregnancy. The ability to communicate across cultural belief systems is essential for this type of research.

Even among members of the majority population are many different belief systems related to health and illness that providers must be aware of. The more we know of the sociocultural diversity within a racial or cultural group, the better able we are not only to provide care but also to determine individuals' willingness to participate in our studies, to ask the right questions, and to undertake the right studies concerning the effect of our care on individual health and function.

Another population aspect that must be considered is access to medical care. Studies will be more representative of the whole community if this access is not limited by socioeconomic or cultural factors, but in the United States many people are under- or uninsured and do not have easy access to public-supported care. The neighborhood health centers that serve poor populations also manage to do a fair amount of practice-based research. The relationship the patients have with the provider and the practice and the role the practice plays in the community affect patient acceptance of practice-based research, regardless of an individual's economic status. Ability to remain in a study may be a particular problem for the poor and for those who have difficulty handling the complexities of daily life, much less these problems posed by the health care system (Clark, 1983).

PAYMENT OF SUBJECTS

In studies that require considerable patient time and commitment or that involve procedures not necessarily sought or needed,

remuneration for the time and inconvenience entailed by participation is important for maintaining continuing involvement.
Obviously, if considerable time, energy, and inconvenience are
incurred and/or there are study-related costs that should not be
borne by the patient, payment becomes essential. Practice-based
research that will lead to profit for others, such as drug trials for
pharmaceutical companies, usually involves payment to the individual patient, or at least free medication.

From my own limited experience, the primary determinant of
participation has been the nature of the study and the relation of
the patients with the individual requesting their participation,
rather than payment.

SOCIAL OR MORAL IMPLICATIONS
OF THE PROBLEM UNDER STUDY,
PUBLIC AWARENESS ATTITUDE, AND
CONFIDENCE IN THE ABILITY OF THE
PRACTICE TO MAINTAIN CONFIDENTIALITY

In some studies, participation may be determined, in part, by
a patient's concern that he or she may be found to have the specific
problem under study and/or whether confidentiality can be
maintained in the practice.

Many ethical issues must be dealt with in conducting any type
of research. In the past, little attention was paid to the importance
of some of these issues. The fact that much confidential material
is dealt with in the patient-provider encounter, as well as the fact
that some research involves the need for active patient understanding of what is being done, requires that all practice-based
research be done in a manner that ensures continued confidentiality in the doctor-patient relationship and minimizes the chance
for any social, psychological, or physical harm befalling the patient
as a result (see Chapter 3). In family practice, confidences affecting the family, as well as the individual, must be considered.
Because many of the employees in a practice may come from the
community served, particularly in small towns, rural areas, and
community-oriented practices anywhere, it is essential that all
staff understand the need to maintain confidentiality about anything learned about individuals cared for in the practice. If the
practice is considered to be the source of leakage of confidential

information into the community, many patients will refuse to seek care unless there are no alternatives, and they will be reluctant to participate in any research projects that require divulging what could be considered to be confidential information.

RETENTION OF PATIENTS
IN PROSPECTIVE STUDIES

One reason some patients enroll in studies is that they believe they will benefit from the extra attention and extra tests. It is important for their continued involvement in a study that this hope be supported. If the patient believes that he or she has lost status as a patient and is seen by the physician only as a study subject, then dissatisfaction will result. Patients seen for scheduled study visits will continue to present other problems that must be either attended to at that time or followed up at an appropriate time.

Conclusion

When the provider-patient relationship is well developed, the study is seen to have value, and the study protocol has minimal impact on usual care, then patient enrollment will proceed well. Family practice patients have responded positively to research in both community and teaching settings.

The organization of the practice can facilitate patient recruitment, particularly the presence of a current age-sex register and morbidity index. It is important not to ignore groups of patients who may appear to be less approachable because of language or culture. Primary care patients, given the appropriate opportunity, have been and will continue to be active participants and partners in research.

References

Beasley, J. W., Cox, N. C., Livingston, B. T., Davis, J. E., Hankey, T. L., Shropshire, R. T., & Roberts, R. G. (1991). Development and operation of the Wisconsin Research Network. *Wisconsin Medical Journal, 90,* 531-537.

Clark, M. M. (1983). Cultural context of medical practice. *Western Journal of Medicine, 139*(6), 806-810.

Green, L. A., Wood, M., Becker, L. A., Farley, E. S., Freeman, W. L., Froom, J., Hames, C., Neibauer, L. J., Rosser, W. W., & Seifert, M. (1984). The ambulatory sentinel practice network: Purpose, methods, and policies. *Journal of Family Practice, 18*(2), 275-280.

Hahn, D., Dodge, R. W., & Golubjatnikov, R. (1991). Association of *Chlamydia pneumoniae* (strain TWAR) and adult-onset asthma. *Journal of the American Medical Association, 266*(2), 225-230.

McDermott, W., Deuschle, K., Adair, J., Fulmer, H., & Loughlin, B. (1960). Introducing modern medicine in a Navajo community. *Science, 131*(3395), 3396, 197-205, 280-287.

Nutting, P. A. (1987). Introduction. In P. A. Nutting (Ed.), *Community-oriented primary care: From principle to practice* (pp. xxi-xxxiii) (Pub. No. HRS-A-PE 86-1). Washington DC: U.S. Department of Health and Human Services.

Wadland, W. C., Hughes, J. R., Secker-Walker, R. H., Bronson, D. L., & Fenwick, J. (1990). Recruitment in a primary care trial on smoking cessation. *Family Medicine, 22*, 201-204.

6   Conducting Qualitative Research in the Practice Setting

JEFFREY M. BORKAN

Introduction

Practice-based qualitative research in primary care is undergoing a growth not experienced previously, with a steady proliferation of studies, investigators, and professional journals. The first task before embarking on it is to ask: What is it and why do it? Add to this a compulsion for answering a question, and the investigatory cycle has begun.

Practice-based research refers to studies conducted in a physician's clinical setting, which comprises patients, staff, colleagues, and community. *Qualitative research* includes a variety of techniques that use interviews and observations, rather than questionnaires or measurements, to generate data. Qualitative research is defined also by its diverse analytical tools, which do not rely on statistics or quantification to arrive at conclusions. Its basis is "non-positivistic," which means that insights are "interpreted," rather than "discovered," and that "truth" is considered to be relative, not absolute. Qualitative research is *inductive*, beginning with observations of reality, formulating insights or understandings, and building theories. In contrast, quantitative investigations are generally *deductive*. They start with theories, construct hypotheses grounded in those theories, and then gather data to support or negate them. In this way, observations often are fitted to prior ideas (Muzzin, 1991).

The qualitative approach emphasizes the importance of *context* in all aspects of an investigation, from conception to dissemination of results. The researcher and the methods are considered to be embedded in the findings, and the concept of *objectivity* is replaced by *reflective subjectivity*. There are no real or symbolic one-way mirrors, and the investigator is always in the picture, influencing everything that is seen and told and serving as an instrument for data collection and analysis (Guba & Lincoln, 1981; McCracken, 1988). The idea, however, is to see as little of the researcher as possible, to leave the subjects adequate leeway to express their stories and ideas. Although often identified with anthropology, qualitative methods are not limited to any one field and may be employed in such diverse disciplines as criminology and health economics.

The incentive for doing practice-based studies, expounded throughout this book, arises from the need to answer a question. This need may start with a clinical problem, a thirst for intellectual stimulation, or a "gut feeling." Research, particularly qualitative research, allows the practitioner to look at the world in a new way—opening the third eye. Such undertakings may reinvigorate the "drab" or reframe the "annoying." If something is arousing anger or frustration, such as noncompliant patients or overly aggressive consultants, it deserves study. Not only is it liable to be a pressing issue in other practices, but also the emotional connection may push the investigation to completion. As Berg, Gordon, and Cherkin (1986) wrote, "Don't get mad, get data" (p. 4). In addition, research improves practice and practice improves research. However, "above all, the search for new knowledge is driven by the intrinsic satisfaction of gaining insight into an important problem and the chance of someday making a difference in the lives of patients" (Berg et al., 1986, p. 2). This difference extends to the lives of communities and societies because health and healing are ultimately social and political.

The most compelling reasons to choose qualitative techniques in practice-based primary care research are contextual: Both the practitioner and the patients are already there, along with their web of questions, problems, and uncertainties. The clinic is a "living laboratory," and the practitioner is ideally placed to observe and inquire. Quantitative studies may be insufficiently sensitive to provide answers to certain questions; qualitative ones may be able to go beyond those limits to gain insights (Blake, 1989; McWilliam, 1992; Willms et al., 1990). For example, a postal survey of asthmatics, using a questionnaire to identify those who experienced stigma, required a qualitative phase to explore meanings and parameters of that experience (Snadden & Brown, 1991). Muzzin (1991) probed the literature on patient referrals before conducting her own study and concluded that only those with a qualitative component contributed to a real understanding of the issue: "Whereas quantitative research counts categories of objects or events, the basic aim of qualitative research is to discover categories or to learn what the instances of a category really *are* (p. 2377).

Questions that lend themselves to qualitative inquiry include Why do patients seek or delay care? What do they do about their condition in addition to soliciting the primary care provider's assistance, including home care or alternative and folk healing? What kinds of explanations do patients (and practitioners) use? What are patients' unexpressed concerns? What is actually happening when they are in the provider's office? What do they understand, and what does the provider understand from what each has told the other? How can the practitioner get a better understanding of disease and health and improve outcomes? What health care practices and unique culture-bound syndromes are common in the population served? How might health care be delivered in a more efficacious and effective manner?

A basic synergy and resonance exist between primary health care (whether family medicine or community nursing) and qualitative research. Both are grounded in the contextual or ecological systems paradigm (Galazka & Eckert, 1986; McWhinney, 1969; Medalie, 1965), and health care providers are natural participant-observers of their practice, their patients, and themselves. The identical logical process operates in qualitative research and clinical medicine, whereby hypotheses or diagnoses are continually revised and refined as new information is *cyclically* collected, interpreted, and analyzed. In both disciplines the direction of the investigation is dependent on the nature of the previous responses. Like the fisherman, the qualitative researcher throws out a broad net of inquiry, pulling and tightening the investigatory mesh with each cycle of questions, observations, and analyses, drawing ever closer to meaningful insights and interpretations. This process departs from standard quantitative exploration, which moves linearly from hypotheses to data collection, and on to analysis and conclusions. In addition, the resonance between qualitative research and primary health care extends to the interviewing process, whereby active listening and a partnership with the patient/informant is sought.

Types of Qualitative Methods and Studies

Innumerable types and combinations of qualitative studies can be conducted in the practice setting. Most, however, fall into three broad categories: participant observation, long interviews, and focus groups. These can be used solely, in conjunction with each other, or with quantitative techniques. Combinations of methods allow the triangulation of data from different sources and can improve the validity and reliability of the study. Qualitative studies are not limited in terms of their design. They may be either prospective or retrospective, observational or experimental.

Participant observation refers to watching while acting—the immersion into a culture in pursuit of understanding from the insider's perspective. Its goal is "to grasp the native's point of view, his relation to life, to realize his vision of the world" (Malinowski, 1922, p. 25). This approach requires repeated and prolonged contact with a community, and its advantages include high authenticity and validity because informants' actions are observed, not just self-reported. Participant observation is useful in circumstances in which having a complete stranger would be an intrusion, both because trust and familiarity can be established and, as time passes, informants are less likely to alter their behavior because of the investigator's presence. In addition to time expenditure, this technique demands intense self-scrutiny because here, more than in any other type of qualitative research, the investigator is the research instrument. Excellent, step-by-step, practical texts for this technique are by Spradley (1980), Bernard (1988), and Bogdewic (1992).

Studies using participant observation as the dominant method vary from reflections on practice to formal fieldwork and are quite common in the primary health literature. At one end of the spectrum are the "rumination" or "philosophical" essays by such thinkers as Ian McWhinney, John Geyman, Jack Medalie, Gayle

Stephens, Lucy Candib, Howard Stein, D. H. Metcalfe, and Joseph Herman, who use their own observations, intuition, and experience to examine issues and to formulate ideas of importance to their discipline. At the other end of the spectrum are examples of more systematic participant observation, as found in studies conducted by Hahn (1985), who looked at the world of an internist; by Katz (1985), on how surgeons make decisions; and by Borkan (1992), on medical risk management in communities. In these reports, lengthy observations were recorded and analyzed carefully by using explicit techniques and full participation in the milieu. In my own example, this participation involved becoming a factory worker in order to observe health and safety activities, not just to hear about them. Here the researcher must understand fully the language and culture of those studied, as well as the sociocultural factors or biases that may impact on the fieldwork situation. Countertransference, or "going native," is a constant threat. For instance, Katz (1985) was horrified to discover that she, like the surgeons she was following, was beginning to recognize patients by their operative sites, rather than by their names.

Long interviews are powerful qualitative tools that focus on specific research questions (Crabtree & Miller, 1991; McCracken, 1988). They vary from unstructured conversations to rigid interview directives and schedules, depending on what information is sought (Miller & Crabtree, 1992), and can generate hypotheses, explore a new area, and take the researcher into the "mental world of the individual, to glimpse the categories and logic by which he or she sees the world" (McCracken, 1988, p. 9). Other advantages include their ability to gather narratives (stories) and to explore sensitive issues requiring self-disclosure—for example, the life experiences of suicide survivors (Van Dongen, 1991) or the full social and psychological ramifications of chronic disease (Kleinman, 1988).

Disadvantages start with the fact that the interviewer can gather information only on what the subject is willing to divulge, and then only the subject's interpretations of actions or events. Interview settings may be highly "decontextualized": They occur apart from what is described, thereby putting further distance between the actual behaviors and the reports of those behaviors. (For this reason, criminal investigators often return with victims or perpetrators to the "scene of the crime.") Narratives in long interviews are dynamic, influenced by the identity of the listener and by the reconstruction of telling and retelling. This activity causes further complications in analysis, which must be considered and overcome.

Long interviews are the basis for the majority of qualitative studies in primary care. There are several reasons for this development: (a) Interviewing is familiar to primary care researchers because it is consonant with the clinical method, (b) both patients and providers are accustomed to and accepting of individual interview situations, (c) recording of interviews is relatively simple, (d) recorded narratives may be transcribed, and (e) uniform analyses may be conducted, thus facilitating comparisons.

Studies vary from single case histories, including those of families (Elhayani, Yechezkel, & Herman, 1991), to examinations of extreme cases, such as instances of cultural blind spots in the physician-patient encounter (Lin, 1983), to elaborate series. In one such case series, Lazarus (1988) followed 53 women throughout their pregnancies and postpartum period, conducting an average of 10 interviews with each. Helman (1978), an English general practitioner and medical anthropologist, examined the relationship between the folk model of "colds and chills" and the local medical model by interviewing a heterogeneous group of patients, nurses, receptionists, and local physicians. There are also numerous examples of medical "storytellers" who document illness narratives from long interviews and clinical interactions, such as Brody (1987), Sacks (1985), and Coles (1989).

Focus group interviewing combines the elements of ethnographic and survey research (Basch, 1987; Bernard, 1988; Morgan, 1988). Through the use of well-defined, prearranged guidelines, groups of individuals are brought together for discussion of a topic, led by a moderator. A wide variety of completed studies exist, including ones on lay persons' perceptions of heart attack risk factors (Morgan & Spanish, 1985), physicians' attitudes toward cancer risk reduction (Valente & Campbell, 1985), and patients' views regarding the efficacy of treatments for low back pain (Cherkin, 1989).

This approach is a relatively new phenomenon in health care research, having been borrowed from its sources in marketing (Merton, Fiske, & Kendall, 1956) and the social sciences. Its strengths include suitability for explorations of a new area, ability to collect rich and diverse experiences, and economy of time and money. Focus groups are able to generate hypotheses, orient the research team to new fields, develop interview schedules and questionnaires, and provide quality control on data collection through the tendency of participants to weed out false information and provide checks and balances (Morgan, 1988; Patton, 1990). They also may generate further interest among participants, afford an enjoyable forum of interaction, and prove therapeutic (Patton, 1990). For instance, in an uncontrolled study, it was found that participants in low back pain focus groups appeared to improve symptomatically (Reis & Borkan, 1991).

The disadvantages of focus groups are similar to those of long interviews. However, this technique has additional difficulties, such as the hesitancy of participants to reveal intimate material, and the potential domination by the majority view.

A comparison of the three methods is displayed in Table 6.1.

How to Get Started

A. CHOOSING A PROBLEM

The qualitative approach to choosing a problem is contextual and reflective. It originates with the interests and needs of the investigator, as well as those of his or her staff, colleagues, patients, and community, and is refined by exploratory data collection, contemplation, and analysis. For instance, I began to investigate psychosocial predictors of back pain after my partners and I had a discussion of our frustrations with treating this ailment. The focus of the study—patient-centered illness models—became apparent only after careful review of the first interviews and observations.

B. SEARCHING THE LITERATURE

In qualitative research, searching a computerized biomedical data base (e.g., Medline) is not enough. Looking only at Index Medicus produces the "I-didn't-find-anything-in-the-literature" syndrome. Escaping such tunnel vision requires entering the world of psychological, sociological, and education searches, which are available at college and university libraries. For instance, searching

Table 6.1 The Three Pillars of Qualitative Research: Choosing a Method of Data Collection

	Participant Observations	*Long Interviews*	*Focus Groups*
Goal	grasp native's point of view	enter the "mental world" of the person	combine survey and ethnographic research
Ideal	examine real behaviors in context	explore specific research questions and gather narratives	generate consensus and unexpected insights
Time	prolonged: days/month	short: hours	short: hours
Economy	low	medium	high
Difficulty	medium-high	low	medium
Reflection of real behavior	very high	variable	variable
Findings influenced by researcher	low-medium	high	medium-high
Suitability for exploration of a new topic	medium-high	high	very high
Help develop questionnaires hypotheses	high	high	high
Data quality control	low	low	high
Elicit intimate or hidden material	medium	high	low
Comfort for researcher	low	high	medium

Medline for literature on the "effects of war" yields almost no citations, but the same exercise in *Psychological Abstracts* reveals a wealth of material, including studies on health effects. Other access points are scholars in a field, texts, and review articles.

C. ASSESSING RESOURCES

Resources, including personal, financial, institutional, and communal, should be assessed early in the planning stage because they will determine the limits of the investigation. Personal resources are based on one's interests, knowledge, and skills, and, of course, time availability. Past experience is relevant, and not only if drawn from anthropological or sociological fieldwork: The skills acquired in any past studies and pursuits where observation, recording, and analysis were important, from journalism to the liberal arts, can be supplemented and put to use. Personal preparation is also essential to foster self-awareness (Bass, 1992).

Finances are generally less of an issue in qualitative research because few instruments and little equipment are required. Expensive items in such work may include research assistant salaries, audio and audiovisual recording equipment, transcription services, computer software, and travel expenses. If the research must be done on a low budget, savings can be achieved by conducting the interviews and observations oneself or with the assistance of colleagues and trainees. Interviews or observations can be recorded on paper or can be audiotaped with the help of dictaphones or cassette recorders fitted with personal or area microphones. Transcription of materials even may be bypassed by analyzing audiotapes or videotapes directly, although this method is impractical with large data sets.

Institutional and community resources include mentors, consultants, collaborators, and support personnel. The community in which one practices may hold hidden resources. For instance, a mentor in research methods could be a clinical psychologist or a member of the humanities faculty of the local community college, and a research team might be assembled from medical or graduate students, local homemakers, and colleagues. I have been amazed at the skills and resources present in whatever community I have worked.

The importance of forming a team cannot be overemphasized. The constant need for reflection, review, and insight may be difficult for the lone investigator; also team members can complement each other's skills and knowledge, aiding the intellectual growth of each participant. Be forewarned, however, that drafting interdisciplinary team members also means acquiring their models and lingos, whether from sociology, psychology, or anthropology.

D. CHOOSING A METHOD
OF DATA COLLECTION

The choice of a data collection method should follow from the
problem being studied and the way the information is communicated. For instance, Newman (1991) discovered that long interviews
were the most appropriate forum for examining physician mistakes because professional self-consciousness precluded open group
discussion, and observations were impractical. A personal "fit"
with the temperament and interests of the researcher is key.
Those who feel comfortable in groups might enjoy focus groups,
while participant observation is appropriate for the contemplative. One qualitative method may lead to another, as Miller (1992)
found in his study of the "routine, ceremony, and drama" of the
family medicine clinic where he practiced. A series of semistruc-
tured key informant interviews spurred him on to participant
observation, taxonomy building, and further long interviews.

E. CHOOSING AN IDENTITY

The clinician undertaking a qualitative study may approach
patients as a health care provider or may choose a specific role
such as investigator, fellow sufferer, or interested third party. The
choice has both ethical and methodological ramifications. For
instance, if you choose to remain the clinician during a long
interview on teenage pregnancy, you limit the range of acceptable
questions (you will have difficulty asking questions that appear
to be clinically irrelevant), whereas taking the role of researcher
creates a relationship that may alter or inhibit future patient-
provider interactions and effectiveness. Finding the proper identity is of equal importance in participant observation or focus
groups. The qualitative approach requires only that the researcher
consider the effects of the chosen approach on the subjects and
information gathered.

F. ETHICAL REVIEW

Ethical issues must be considered, whether in protecting your
informants, dealing with institutional review boards, or examining your own biases. Examples of problems include sensitive

data collection (as with rape victims or drug abusers), political considerations (as in studying AIDS patients or victims of torture), or undue identification with your subjects ("going native"). Informed consent, difficult enough in long interviews and focus groups, enters uncharted waters when considered in the context of participant observation. These issues are discussed in Chapter 3 and by Punch (1986).

G. CHOOSING A SITE AND GAINING ACCESS

Site choice may be one of convenience, such as the primary health clinic or hospital in which you practice, or a directed choice aimed at maximizing observational or interviewing possibilities. For instance, it probably would be more fruitful to study high-risk behaviors for AIDS associated with illicit drug use at a methadone clinic rather than at a suburban family practice. The choice of a site will permeate all aspects of the research, including the generalizability of the findings.

Gaining access is often a project in itself because personnel at many settings are wary of allowing outsiders close inspection of their operations. Will your partners, patients, and local hospital allow you to scrutinize clinical interactions, "rounds," or board meetings? In gaining access, discussions with the managing institution are helpful, as are appeals to the right persons in the organization's hierarchy. (During my Ph.D. fieldwork, I was faced with disaster when the comparison industrial site was suddenly closed to me by the local factory boss. I appealed my way up the corporate ladder until I discovered a sympathetic vice president who had a son studying for his doctorate, and the doors reopened.)

H. GOING TO THE FIELD

The start of *fieldwork*—the data collection phase of the investigation—begins with the first casual observations. This part may involve looking afresh at your own practice or visiting farmers in their agricultural setting.

The end of fieldwork usually is reached when you believe that you understand the material as well as your subjects do, and you cease to uncover new insights or information.

I. RECORDING

Qualitative fieldwork requires more than interviews and observations. Careful, systematic recording is also of critical importance. Whether the mechanics involve written, audio, or video recordings, the rule of thumb is that as little time as possible should pass between the event and its chronicling. Special software programs exist for text management and hypothesis generation, and these can be helpful in analysis (Fielding & Lee, 1991; Tesch, 1990).

Records of observations should relate to both content and process, with each aspect coded separately. These records might be supplemented by a fieldwork diary that reflects on the emotive side of research. (Occasionally these diaries come to be more interesting than the work itself, and several classic ones have been published.)

J. ANALYZING

The key to qualitative analysis is immersion in the data until you learn to speak with the same voice as those you study, having come to understand their world from the inside. A critical part of the qualitative research cycle of "data collection → analysis → conclusions → data collection" is early and repeated review of your findings with informants, colleagues, "blinded" judges, and mentors. Insights can be used to refine the interview questions and to improve the validity of the study because initial findings and conjectures can be returned to the field for retesting. In a 3-year study of hip fractures (Borkan, Quirk, & Sullivan, 1991), we achieved this refinement through the use of frequent "retreats" by the research team; reviews of sample transcripts by outside consultants; discussions with therapists, nurses, and physicians involved in patient care; and written feedback by transcriptionists. This process led to constant refinements of the research techniques and our conclusions.

Analytical strategies in qualitative research are as diverse as the issues studied. They can be seen, however, as stretching along a continuum from the objective, scientific, deductive, technical, and standardized, to the subjective, intuitive, inductive, context-dependent, and interpretive (Miller & Crabtree, 1992). At one extreme are methods such as "immersion-crystallization," prolonged study, and reflection on a text until intuitive themes emerge (Miller & Crabtree, 1992); at the other extreme are statistical manipulations of data sets (Miles & Huberman, 1984; Tesch, 1990). As with choosing methods of data collection, the analytical tools should be consistent with the issue and with the researcher's inclinations. For instance, those who favor the broad overview might feel more comfortable searching for dominant themes, while more exacting researchers might prefer the micro-world of linguistic analysis, examining word choices and syntax (Mishler, 1984; Weber, 1990). Special techniques exist for the analysis of audiotapes and videotapes (Stewart, 1992).

K. DISSEMINATION AND FEEDBACK

In practice-based qualitative research, the researcher has the responsibility to disseminate information back to the "community" (staff, professional colleagues, and the practice area) and should discuss with subjects how the investigation can be useful and communicated to them. For instance, in a focus group and long interview study of low back pain, some participants requested a lecture on the subject at a later time, while others asked for a copy of the manuscript (Reis & Borkan, 1991). Dissemination also may involve introducing improvements in diagnosis and therapeutics, educational materials, articles (both lay and professional), and health care training seminars. In one study, findings that were generated from focus groups of family physicians on the issue of identification and treatment of wife abuse served as a guide in the development of three workshops for clinical practitioners on this subject (Brown, Lent, & Sas, 1992).

A Summary of Suggestions

A. In practice-based research, the questions are all around you. Be open to research ideas and opportunities, keep a log, and start with the questions that compel you.

B. The research begins when the first question is asked or the first observation is made. Throw out a broad net of inquiry and carefully

pull it in. Immerse yourself in the data until you and the inform-
ants speak with the same voice.
C. *The less seen of the researcher the better.* In qualitative work, the
    researcher and interviewer should have minimal roles, leaving
    space for the voices and experiences of the subjects.
D. *Protect your subjects.* You have special ethical responsibilities in
    qualitative research to protect confidentiality and consider po-
    tential impact.
E. *The rule of resonance.* The process of qualitative research should
    resonate with clinical work. Attempt to make the research syner-
    gistic with other aspects of your professional and personal life,
    rather than let it detract from them.
F. *Collaboration.* Get a team of collaborators involved early, drawing
    from your own or other fields. Be prepared to go outside your
    discipline in seeking literature, advice, or collaboration. There is
    a mentor, teacher, or assistant around every corner. Get feedback
    at every turn.
G. *Enjoy yourself.* Research should be fun as well as enlightening.

References

Basch, C. E. (1987). Focus group interview: An underutilized research technique
    for improving theory and practice in health education. *Health Education Quar-
    terly, 14,* 411-418.
Bass, M. J. (1992). The clinician in research: Identifying questions and observing.
    In M. Stewart, F. Tudiver, M. J. Bass, E. V. Dunn, & P. G. Norton (Eds.), *Tools for
    primary care research* (pp. 29-35). Newbury Park, CA: Sage.
Berg, A. O., Gordon, M. J., & Cherkin, D. C. (1986). *Practice-based research in family
    medicine.* Kansas City, MO: Burd & Fletcher.
Bernard, H. R. (1988). *Research methods in cultural anthropology.* Newbury Park,
    CA: Sage.
Blake, R. L. (1989). Integrating quantitative and qualitative methods in family
    research. *Family Systems Medicine, 7*(4), 411-427.
Bogdewic, S. P. (1992). Participant observation. In B. F. Crabtree & W. L. Miller (Eds.),
    Doing qualitative research in primary care (pp. 45-69). Newbury Park, CA: Sage.
Borkan, J. M. (1992). Risk management in the community: Lesson for family
    medicine. *Family Practice, 9*(1), 42-48.
Borkan, J. M., Quirk, M., & Sullivan, M. (1991). After the fall: Injury narratives of
    elderly hip fracture patients. *Social Science and Medicine, 33*(8), 947-957.
Brody, H. (1987). *Stories of sickness.* New Haven, CT: Yale University Press.
Brown, J. B., Lent, B., & Sas, G. (1992, April). *The use of focus groups to identify the
    problems and solutions encountered by family physicians in the identification and
    treatment of wife abuse.* Paper presented at the Annual Meeting of the North
    American Primary Care Research Group, Richmond, VA.

Cherkin, D. L. (1989). Patient evaluations of low back pain care from family physicians and chiropractors. *Western Journal of Medicine, 150,* 351-355.

Coles, R. (1989). *The call of stories.* Boston: Houghton Mifflin.

Crabtree, B. F., & Miller, W. L. (1991). A qualitative approach to primary care research: The long interview. *Family Medicine, 23*(2), 145-151.

Elhayani, A., Yechezkel, A., & Herman, J. (1991). Paradigm lost: Cross-cultural considerations in a patient with panic attacks. *Family Systems Medicine, 9*(2), 165-170.

Fielding, N. G., & Lee, R. M. (Eds.). (1991). *Using computers in qualitative research.* Newbury Park, CA: Sage.

Galazka, S. S., & Eckert, J. K. (1986). Clinically applied anthropology: Concepts for the family physician. *Journal of Family Practice, 22,* 159-165.

Guba, E. G., & Lincoln, Y. S. (1981). *Effective evaluations.* San Francisco: Jossey-Bass.

Hahn, R. A. (1985). A world of internal medicine: Portrait of an internist. In R. A. Hahn & A. D. Gaines (Eds.), *Physicians of Western medicine* (pp. 51-111). Dordrecht, The Netherlands: D. Reidel.

Helman, C. G. (1978). "Feed a cold, starve a fever": Folk models of infection in an English suburban community, and their relation to medical treatment. *Culture, Medicine and Psychiatry, 2,* 107-137.

Katz, P. (1985). How surgeons make decisions. In R. A. Hahn & A. D. Gaines (Eds.), *Physicians of Western medicine* (pp. 155-175). Dordrecht, The Netherlands: D. Reidel.

Kleinman, A. (1988). *The illness narratives.* New York: Basic Books.

Lazarus, E. S. (1988). Theoretical considerations for the study of the doctor-patient relationship: Implications of a perinatal study. *Medical Anthropology Quarterly, 2*(1), 34-58.

Lin, E. H. (1983). Intraethnic characteristics and the patient-physician interaction: "Cultural blind spot syndrome." *Journal of Family Practice, 16*(1), 91-98.

Malinowski, B. (1922). *Argonauts of the Western Pacific.* London: Routledge.

McCracken, G. (1988). *The long interview.* Newbury Park, CA: Sage.

McWhinney, I. R. (1969). The foundations of family medicine. *Canadian Family Physician, 4,* 13-27.

McWilliam, C. L. (1992). From hospital to home: The elderly's discharge experience. *Family Medicine, 24*(6), 457-468.

Medalie, J. H. (1965). Levels of practice. *Journal of the College of General Practice, 9,* 20-43.

Merton, R. K., Fiske, M., & Kendall, P. L. (1956). *The focused interview.* New York: Free Press.

Miles, M. S., & Huberman, A. M. (1984). *Qualitative data analysis: A sourcebook of new methods.* Beverly Hills, CA: Sage.

Miller, W. L. (1992). Routine, ceremony, or drama: An exploratory field study of the primary care clinical encounter. *Journal of Family Practice, 34*(3), 289-296.

Miller, W. L., & Crabtree, B. F. (1992). Primary care research: A multi-method typology and qualitative road map. In B. F. Crabtree & W. L. Miller (Eds.), *Doing qualitative research in primary care* (pp. 3-28). Newbury Park, CA: Sage.

Mishler, E. G. (1984). *The discourse of medicine: Dialectics of medical interviews.* Norwood, NJ: Ablex.

Morgan, D. L. (1988). *Focus groups as qualitative research.* Newbury Park, CA: Sage.

Morgan, D. L., & Spanish, M. T. (1985). Social interaction and the cognitive organization of health-relevant behavior. *Sociology of Health and Illness, 7,* 401-422.

Muzzin, L. (1991). Understanding the process of medical referral. *Canadian Family Physician, 37,* 2377-2382.

Newman, M. (1991). *The emotional impact of mistakes upon family physicians.* Paper presented at the Annual Meeting of the North American Primary Care Research Group, Quebec City, Quebec.

Patton, M. (1990). *Qualitative evaluation and research methods.* Newbury Park, CA: Sage.

Punch, M. (1986). *The politics and ethics of fieldwork.* Beverly Hills, CA: Sage.

Reis, S., & Borkan, J. M. (1991). *Talking about the pain: An analysis of focus groups on low back pain.* Paper presented at the Annual Meeting of the North American Primary Care Research Group, Quebec City, Quebec.

Sacks, O. (1985). *The man who mistook his wife for a hat and other clinical tales.* New York: Summit.

Snadden, D., & Brown, J. B. (1991). Asthma and stigma. *Family Practice, 8,* 329-334.

Spradley, J. P. (1980). *Participant observation.* New York: Holt, Rinehart & Winston.

Stewart, M. (1992). Approaches to audiotape and videotape analysis. In B. F. Crabtree & W. L. Miller (Eds.), *Doing qualitative research in primary care* (pp. 149-162). Newbury Park, CA: Sage.

Tesch, R. (1990). *Qualitative research: Analysis types and software tools.* New York: Falmer.

Valente, C. M., & Campbell, Y. L. (1985). Cancer risk reduction: A focus on physicians. *Maryland Medical Journal, 34,* 67-70.

Van Dongen, C. J. (1991). Experiences of family members after a suicide. *Journal of Family Practice, 33*(4), 375-380.

Weber, R. P. (1990). *Basic content analysis* (2nd ed.). Newbury Park, CA: Sage.

Willms, D. G., Best, J. A., Taylor, D. W., Gilbert, J. R., Wilson, D. M. C., Lindsay, E. A., & Singer, J. (1990). A systematic approach for using qualitative methods in primary prevention research. *Medical Anthropology Quarterly, 4,* 391-409.

7   Realizing the Research Potential of the Office Computer

WILLIAM E. HOGG
JACQUES LEMELIN

Computerization of the office is a critically important preparation to organizing a research practice. Too often the office computer is used only for billing, its research potential unrecognized. In this chapter we describe alternative ways of collecting clinical data, discuss their impact on cost and on data integrity, and identify characteristics of electronic record systems that can aid office research. We also suggest questions to ask when investigating the research capability of a medical record computer system. To illustrate the issues discussed here, we present three examples of office-based research made possible because of computerized medical records.

The field of family practice is rich, and we believe that every practice has special characteristics that deserve to be the focus of research. The first step is to identify these characteristics. For example, our family practice was in Wakefield, a small town near Ottawa, composed of a mixed French- and English-speaking population. The six doctors provided almost all of the care for this stable community—in the office, home, emergency department, and hospital.

The next step is to decide which baseline information you want to record so that, in the future, research will be facilitated. Because most research using these data will be cross-sectional or descriptive cohort studies, you should record data on potential confounding variables, as well as information that might help you track down patients who move.

Having decided on the type of data you want to collect, the next questions are How much will it cost? and How should it be collected? To address these issues, we will proceed by presenting research study examples, chosen to portray a broad range of data elements and types of research, and to make certain points about basic data requirements in office-based research. These examples have not been chosen for their clinical relevance or for their generalizability to other practices: Each reflects one or more of the special characteristics of our particular setting and may not transfer directly to other settings. Remember, it is precisely because of the rich differences between practices that the practice is a special place for research.

Study 1
Preventive Medicine Reminder Letter Study

One of the authors (Hogg, 1990) was principal investigator of a randomized controlled trial aimed at increasing patient compliance with preventive health measures. The goal here was to evaluate the cost-effectiveness of computer-generated family-oriented reminder letters sent out to patients.

This study exploited several special characteristics of the Wakefield practice setting: intact families, a stable population, and the fact that most people in the area attend the one group of doctors.

DATA ELEMENTS

Language of the recipients had to be known here so that letters could be sent in either English or French. To adjust for the potentially confounding effects of poverty, the parents' number of years of education and most recent occupation were collected as indicators of socioeconomic class. The data base also had to keep track of the dates and ordering of the preventive procedures, the dates that the letters were sent out, and whether a patient was in the intervention or control group.

DATA INTEGRITY, COLLECTION
ALTERNATIVES, AND COST

Language, number of years of education, and occupation data
were collected by the same automated demographic updating
system described on page 92. The cost for maintaining all of the
registration data was 8 cents per patient per year.
The preventive procedures followed in the study included
DPTP #1-5, TOPV, MMR, H. influenza, dT, tetanus toxoid, MMR
booster, Rubella screen, Pap, mammogram, hemoccult, flu shots,
pneumovax, and cholesterol. In our practice, when a procedure
is ordered or given, the physician circles that procedure on a paper
data collection sheet (Hogg, 1990; North, 1989) and this information, along with that required for government medical insurance
billing, is input later into the computer system. It takes only a
second or two of time and pays off because the updated computer
file resulting from each encounter will prompt the doctor for all
overdue preventive procedures. In the long run, this procedure
saves time for the doctor and improves care.

QUESTIONS FOR THE VENDOR

Conducting such a study requires software that identifies
whether a patient is eligible for each preventive procedure, checks
when that patient last had the procedure, and determines whether
this date falls within prescribed time intervals (whether the patient is overdue). It then integrates this information with word-
processing files so that personalized letters can be composed. Ask
the vendor whether patient-specific data can be incorporated
into letters.
This project also requires a sophistication in analysis beyond
that normally possessed by practicing physicians, so it may be
necessary to extract data onto floppy disks and send these to an
outside consultant statistician. Ask the vendor whether the system has a data export capability.
Check that the system provides accessory fields to use in keeping
track of the different intervention groups and mailing dates.
(Most, if not all, systems will have such a feature.)

Study 2
Influence of Setting on Prescribing Pattern

Our next example describes a study that compared medication prescribing patterns of physicians in two different settings: the office and the emergency room. In a retrospective study, the behavior of each of six physicians was looked at in both of these settings. We selected four common illnesses that should present at similar stages of severity in each setting and, to make the conditions as comparable as possible, restricted each medical condition to a particular gender and age grouping. It was found that all doctors prescribed substantially more frequently for the same illness when in the emergency room.

(This study exploited the special characteristic that all of the doctors at the Wakefield hospital also worked in the nearby private office and that competing medical services are relatively inaccessible.)

DATA ELEMENTS

Data elements required by this study were the setting, the physician, the diagnosis, all medication prescribed at that visit, the postal code (to ensure only local residents were included), the date of the visit, and the patient's age and gender.

DATA INTEGRITY, COLLECTION
ALTERNATIVES, AND COST

All of these variables, except diagnosis and prescription data, are required for billing the provincial insurance plan. Therefore no extra cost was involved, and the data should be complete and reliable. Collection of the two nonstandard data elements is discussed below.

Diagnosis

Although government insurance agencies require a diagnosis, it is not necessary or routine to provide accurate diagnostic information. Furthermore the government requires only one diagnosis to process a bill, even if the physician has dealt with several problems.

The accuracy of the diagnostic information depends primarily on the physician's commitment to having complete and accurate data (Dambro & Weiss, 1988; Payne, Goroll, Morgan, & Barnett, 1990). This assignment is best achieved when the physician uses those data on a regular basis as part of clinical care. This use is accomplished when the computer provides a report that summarizes the patient's medical history in a useful, convenient, and up-to-date fashion (O'Keefe-Whiting, Simborg, Epstein, & Warger, 1985).

In many offices (North, 1989), doctors write the diagnosis on a paper form, and a trained data entry clerk then translates this to a coding system. Dambro and Weiss (1988) found the main reason for errors in this type of system was poor handwriting that had been improperly interpreted by the clerks. A policy whereby the clerk marked difficult words, with subsequent review by the physician, improved the error rate substantially. Having the doctor write the diagnosis and a clerk do the coding, in our opinion, is still the preferred method. We believe that having physicians do their own coding would slow them down, which is incompatible with good data, as well as having significant financial impact on the practice.

Some centers have the doctors do the coding and the clerk input the already-coded data. On the face of it, this second method seems to offer better data integrity, but there is a tendency for doctors to overuse the few codes that they have committed to memory. With the "look up" capability of modern microcomputers, the clerk can do the coding and data entry in virtually the same time as just the data entry alone. (A discussion of classifications for primary care is found in Wood [1992, in Volume 2 of this series].)

Prescription Data

To have the comprehensive and accurate drug data required by this study, the collection method must be physician friendly, and it must be possible for the computer to manipulate the information to serve the doctors in their daily practice. Collection methods that take up the physicians' time will be expensive and unacceptable. One option is to use a pressure-sensitive duplicate prescription section as part of the form the doctor fills out for data collection and the computer summary report. The computer fills in the date and the patient's name and address, which saves possibly a few seconds; the doctor then writes the prescription, signs it, tears off a detachable portion, gives this to the patient, and is left with a duplicate of the prescription still attached to the data collection form. Other data collection alternatives, including direct entry by the physician, will not be discussed here.

QUESTIONS FOR THE VENDOR

The system must have a statistical query module that allows extraction of *all* elements of the data base (Barnett, 1984; McDonald & Tierney, 1986; Payne et al., 1990).

Ask for a demonstration in which you set the terms of the question. A sample question: Could I obtain a list of all male patients aged 15 to 25 years with alcoholism? Usually at exhibits or demonstrations the vendors have added only 100 or so patient files to their demo equipment. No wonder it works and is fast. Speak directly with a customer to find out how well it works in the field. Is it user friendly? Does it have error detection as data are put in? Does it have an on-screen help function? Is statistics training included in the price, and is help included in the software maintenance? Can the research statistics module be password-protected so that access can be restricted to only certain members of the office? Can several research queries on the same file be batched together for efficiency? Are error messages understandable to the average user?

Ask how the system uses diagnostic and prescription information to help doctors in their day-to-day practice of clinical medicine (Hogg, 1990). Request an example of the computer summary sheet, and check to see how it tracks patients' permanent problems, immunizations, risk factors, allergies, family history, current medications, and so on. If the data are packaged in a form that the clinician uses, he or she can ensure the data are accurate and complete. Is the data collection system doctor friendly?

Study Idea:
Earlier Diagnosis of Family Crisis

Illness occurs more frequently when people are stressed (McWhinney, 1989). For example, when one member of a family is tense and struggling, other members may consult their doctor for conditions that they otherwise would have coped with themselves (Balint, 1964). The psychosocial conflict may not be recognized by such patients as contributing to their illness and help-seeking behavior. Not all people choose to confide psychosocial difficulties with their doctor; thus the doctor may be unaware of the family crisis and may order expensive, unnecessary, or potentially dangerous tests and medications with resulting delays in diagnosis, which may affect the prognosis. Noticing an increase in the visitation rate may be a doctor's first indication of a problem. However, members of the family may present after regular hours and see several different doctors of a group practice, making it difficult for the personal physician to notice the increased rate of visitation. These thoughts led us to consider a study that would test the existence of this phenomenon and whether increasing the doctor's awareness was of value.

A computer system could be programmed to calculate a baseline visitation rate for a family unit over several years and to compare it against the visitation rate over the previous 3-month period. Automatically performing this calculation for each appointment, the computer would alert the doctor if a marked increase in the visitation rate had occurred. The study objective would be to determine whether this prompt helped the doctor diagnose important problems earlier.

This study would exploit several characteristics of the Wakefield practice setting, including the intact families, a stable population, the grouping of all physicians in the same practice, and a comprehensive data base made possible by the integration of emergency room visits and office visits in the same data base. Settings without these characteristics would not be able to undertake this specific research.

DATA ELEMENTS

Two data elements required for this study are the date of each encounter for each family member and a link between family members.

DATA INTEGRITY, COLLECTION
ALTERNATIVES, AND COST

The date of each encounter is collected routinely for Canadian medical billing purposes, which ensures its completeness and accuracy. Thus no extra cost is associated with its collection that can be attributed to the research, other than the extra computer memory required when data are kept long after billing is completed.

Many computer systems come with the ability to link families together (Calman, Harvey, & Shah, 1982; Schneeweiss, 1990) and update registration data, so there is usually no extra charge for this software enhancement. In the automated system in Wakefield (Hogg & Crouch, in press), the computer data base is tied to the appointment scheduler and generates household information reports that are given to the patients for updating as they attend. This procedure ensures accurate information for the entire family. Only changes or new data need be input to the data base. The cost of maintaining the demographic data base, including the extra data that reflect the special characteristics of the practice in Wakefield, is 8 cents per patient per year. The initial cost to register a patient and establish the family linkage was 36 cents per patient.

QUESTIONS FOR THE VENDOR

If you were to attempt such a study, you would require a long-term data base so that the software algorithm used to prompt the doctor could access data going back several years. Family doctors trying to set up a general research capability will not have settled in advance all of the research projects they might ever want to do. If some data elements are deleted routinely, research options are lost. It is best, therefore, that as much data as possible be kept indefinitely. A good question to ask a computer salesperson is, Is the data base purged periodically when the accounts have been reconciled, or can all data elements that are entered be stored indefinitely?

Ask whether there is an automated demographic updating system. Can the mechanism link families? Is it linked to an appointment scheduler so that the same information does not have to be entered twice?

Finally, to conduct this study, the computer needs the ability to alert the doctors to the issue of interest (Barnett, 1984; McDonald & Tierney, 1986; North, 1989). Using software algorithms, it must be able to produce, either on paper or on screen, a report that provides clinically useful information. The prompts must be helpful, or else the doctor will ignore them.

Discussion

These three study examples show the complexity of research that could be carried out in a practice setting to exploit the special characteristics of that setting. Most of the data elements already are required for billing purposes, and, therefore, their collection does not involve extra cost. The routine collection of additional data elements should be proven to either save the physician time or enhance quality of care, in order to be justified. The data collection system should be integrated as much as possible with the billing: Physicians can only sustain motivation to collect accurate and comprehensive data when their billing or day-to-day clinical care depends on it. Every effort must be made not to slow down the doctor in the name of research. Be skeptical if a salesperson tells you that a system was designed initially to do research and only later made to incorporate billing.

Few MDs will choose a computer system for an office solely on its capacity to do research. Nonetheless, if a system includes this ability, it opens the door to great possibilities.

The Future Role of Computers

Computers are increasing in power and decreasing in price at an astonishing pace that seems only to accelerate. Their affordability and ubiquity mean that the knowledge and skills needed to run and maintain them are becoming widespread. Increasingly medical students are receiving training in medical informatics as part of their education (Bresnitz, Stettin, & Gabrielson, 1986; Protti, 1989).

Medical office computer software is becoming more sophisticated as the commercial sector progresses in a competitive marketplace, and clinical applications soon may be so compelling that it no longer will be possible to practice medicine to an acceptable standard without the help of computers. Links to the laboratory and to real time drug expert systems are only two of the many exciting areas certain to be widespread relatively soon. The ability to dictate text directly into the computer will change medical records in a revolutionary manner: With the development of speaker-independent voice-recognition software capable of recognizing 5,000 to 20,000 words, computer systems for various specialties and family medicine are being developed (Halbrook, 1991), and some are already in use (Cass, 1991). Soon family physicians will be able to enter verbally all clinical data for a fraction of the cost of a full-time secretary and data entry clerk.

The methods for network research are maturing (Iverson, Calonge, Miller, Niebauer, & Reed, 1988), while data standards for computer medical records are emerging. These two developments could collide, with enormous impact for family medicine. Computerized networks with data from millions of patients might soon be a reality—and a research gold mine. Inexpensive memory and powerful processors make it feasible to keep data indefinitely. Grouping together practices with similar characteristics will provide power to examine even low-prevalence problems in detail, while practices with different characteristics offer opportunities for comparison.

The need for community-based research is well established (Hogg, 1991), as practicing physicians are ideally positioned to know what areas most urgently require information and study. Although doctors may experience difficulties doing research, they also will benefit enormously (Bass, 1987; Hogg, 1991). Indications are that government policy will place an increasing emphasis on community-based care (Gerstein et al., 1991), and research funding eventually should shift to be more available to primary care disciplines and community-based physicians.

We have stressed our opinion that computerization of the office plays an important part in creating a research infrastructure. Today's computers and medical software industry are already able to provide an effective infrastructure to allow office-based research, and we are optimistic that future developments will offer even more rewards. Many important research projects can and have been done in office practice without computers. But if you are going to computerize anyway, why not ensure this potential?

References

Balint, M. (1964). *The doctor, his patient and the illness* (2nd ed.). Toronto: Pitman.

Barnett, G. O. (1984). The application of computer-based medical record systems in ambulatory practice. *New England Journal of Medicine, 310,* 1643-1650.

Bass, M. (1987). Office-based research: The antidote to learned helplessness. *Canadian Family Physician, 33,* 1987-1992.

Bresnitz, E. A., Stettin, G. D., & Gabrielson, I. W. (1986). A survey of computer literacy among medical students. *Journal of Medical Education, 61,* 410-412.

Calman, N., Harvey, M., & Shah, R. (1982). A computerized family problem profile. *Family Practice Research Journal, 2*(1), 63-72.

Cass, O. (1991, November). *Voice GI.* Presented at the Fifth Annual Symposium on Computer Applications in Medical Care, Washington, DC.

Dambro, M. R., & Weiss, B. D. (1988). Assessing the quality of data entry in a computerized medical records system. *Journal of Medical Systems, 12*(3), 181-187.

Gerstein, R., Labelle, J., MacLeod, S., Mustard, F., Spasoff, R., & Watson, J. (1991). Nurturing health: A framework on the determinants of health. In *Premier's Council on Health Strategy* (pp. 1-32). Toronto: Premier's Council.

Halbrook, J. (1991, November). *Emergency medicine (voice EM).* Presented at the Fifth Annual Symposium on Computer Applications in Medical Care, Washington, DC.

Hogg, W. (1990). The role of computers in preventive medicine in a rural family practice. *Canadian Medical Association Journal, 143*(1), 33-37.

Hogg, W. (1991). A community-based practice as a research laboratory, Part 2: Combining practice and research. *Canadian Family Physician, 37,* 2357-2359.

Hogg, W., & Crouch, H. (in press). Incorporating the family into a computerized medical record. *Family Medicine.*

Iverson, D. C., Calonge, B. N., Miller, R. S., Niebauer, L. J., & Reed, F. M. (1988). The development and management of a primary care network. *Family Medicine, 20,* 177-180.

McDonald, C. J., & Tierney, M. D. (1986). Research uses of computer stored practice records in general medicine. *Journal of General Internal Medicine, 4*(Suppl. July-August), S19-24.

McWhinney, I. R. (1989). *A textbook of family medicine.* New York: Oxford University Press.

North, J. (1989). Use an encounter sheet to solve your problems. *Australian Family Physician, 18*(1), 26-28.

O'Keefe-Whiting, Q. E., Simborg, D. W., Epstein, W. V., & Warger, A. (1985). A computerized summary medical record system can provide more information than the standardized medical record. *Journal of the American Medical Association, 254*(9), 1185-1192.

Payne, T. H., Goroll, A. H., Morgan, M., & Barnett, G. O. (1990). Conducting a matched-pairs historical cohort study with a computer-based ambulatory medical record system. *Computers and Biomedical Research, 23,* 455-472.

Protti, D. J. (1989). The status of medical informatics in Canadian medical schools. *Methods of Information in Medicine, 28,* 223-226.

Schneeweiss, R. (1990). An opposing view. *Journal of Family Practice, 30*(6), 700-703.

Wood, M. (1992). The international classification of primary care. In M. Stewart, F. Tudiver, M. J. Bass, E. V. Dunn, & P. G. Norton (Eds.), *Tools for primary care research* (pp. 36-49). Newbury Park, CA: Sage.

8 Identifying and Responding to Community Needs

BRIAN MORRIS
GIORA ALMAGOR

Introduction

As a community-based family physician, my (Morris) personal research efforts have been centered around the needs of my own community of Barrie, Ontario, a city of 50,000. In this setting I have examined the seroprevalence of hepatitis B in our local sexually transmitted diseases clinic and have found it to be much lower than in large urban centers (Morris, Harason, & Butler-Jones, 1992). I have looked at different ways of encouraging schoolchildren to wear bicycle helmets and have used local resources to find ways that work in my community (Morris & Trimble, 1991). I also have addressed myself to the needs (as I perceived them) of other communities within my practice.

All of this, however, has been done on an informal basis. I have never rigorously assessed the needs of any of "my" communities. I have not even gone through the steps of defining those communities, nor have I studied whether my work has been of use to the people in them. In fact, until I started to prepare for the conference that led to this book, I was not even aware that a formal, comprehensive system existed for "identifying and responding to community needs."

In this chapter we examine some of the theory and methods involved in carrying out primary care research based on the model of community oriented primary care (COPC). The COPC approach encompasses a set of principles and techniques that allow medical practitioners to define, study, and organize a practice along community lines (Nutting, 1987). Integral to a COPC practice are a number of research-based steps. These steps are the focus of this chapter. In a postscript, Dr. Giora Almagor describes how this process has been applied in an urban practice in Israel.

Applying COPC in Practice

The first step is to come up with a definition and description of a particular "community." Depending on context, these can vary from an age/sex register of a solo practice to a sophisticated survey of a region's economic and health status, examining such factors as the demand, supply, and capacity of primary care resources (Hogg, 1984). Denominator problems are addressed and a community diagnosis can be made.

The second step is to identify community health problems, whether examining global issues or specific problems of interest to the researcher, a funding agency, or the community. Techniques used here include group processes and "microepidemiology."

Once problems have been identified, the third step is to formulate a response. This response may involve health promotion, treatment of a medical problem, or reorganization of a healthcare facility. In addition to clinical activities, the physician may be involved as an advocate (Morris & Butler-Jones, 1991) or a role model. The fourth and final step is to study the impact of any intervention.

Each of these steps requires research techniques—and not always conventional biomedical ones. Understanding and using the COPC model and principles will give community physicians a framework within which their efforts can be placed.

DEFINING THE COMMUNITY

The dictionary definition of *community* is of limited use here. To know that a community is "a body of people living near one another and in a social relationship . . . with a faith, profession, or way of life in common" (*New Webster's Dictionary and Thesau-*

rus of the English Language, 1991, p. 198) does not help much. It may be simpler to think of a community as any identifiable group of people with some common characteristic. For instance, a *practice community* (Hawk & Calvert, 1987) can be defined as the active patients in a practice. This population shares the common characteristic of having the same doctor and is a group with which the practitioner can identify easily. To offer health care (existing and new programs) and to assume responsibility for the members of this community is a concept that most physicians would be comfortable with.

Then the subgroups within the practice community will each have their own common characteristics and special needs and appropriately could be considered as separate communities (although some might think of these as cohorts). A subgroup might consist, say, of people with a particular disease—for example, diabetes. These individuals, when described as the "community of people in my practice with diagnosed diabetes," can readily be seen to have special needs with regard to regular follow-up, specialist involvement, vaccination against influenza, and so on. Similar subgroups within a practice might be based on risk factors (e.g., smokers), age (the elderly), employment (high-risk jobs or *lack* of employment), ethnic background (association with certain genetic diseases or with health beliefs that conflict with those of the physician), or any other medical or demographic factor. In all of these situations, the definition of *community* can lead to opportunities within one's practice both for research and for better patient care.

All of these factors also can be used to define communities outside of a single practice. Two examples come to mind from my personal experience. In Barrie, government funding recently has been awarded to a group of family doctors, public health workers, educators, and lay people to improve neonatal morbidity and mortality by focusing on the health of a specific local "community": pregnant women. In this example, the community already has been defined, its health needs assessed, and a program established. Similarly, in the work I did with the "community of Barrie schoolchildren who ride bicycles" to encourage them to wear helmets, the population was defined on the basis of age, a common risk factor, and the need for a specific intervention. In sum, the definition of *community* can be based on any relevant factors and can be enlarged to any size that can be handled (practice, hospital, city, region, province, country).

How is research involved in defining a community? In numerous ways. It is often required simply to identify the members of the community. How many diabetics do I really have in my practice? A literature search will help first with the diagnostic criteria for diabetes; a practice audit then will determine what proportion of my practice have had a screening test; and a cross-sectional study may be required to identify accurately all diabetics.

Epidemiologic methods involving census data (Galazka & Zyzanski, 1987) can be used to compare a practice community to a larger population (a city or province). This comparison is necessary if one wishes to generalize from one's own practice.

IDENTIFYING COMMUNITY NEEDS

Once the first step has been taken of defining a community—whether it be large or small, practice based, or diagnosis based—the next step is to decide on the *needs*, the *health problems*, of that community. A variety of methods is available to do this, ranging from the simple (or simplistic!) to the sophisticated.

The simplest way to identify health problems is to do it yourself. What conditions are being poorly treated in your practice? What facilities are lacking in your area? What preventable diseases are still common? This contemplative approach may be a good starting point for a more detailed inquiry.

A logical next step would be to involve a group—of other physicians, other health care professionals, or other "stakeholders." This is the approach we used when doing our bicycle helmet work: We invited teachers, police safety officers, service clubs, public health officials, retailers, racers, parents—everyone we could think of. By seeking a broad spectrum of ideas and approaches, we greatly increased the likelihood that our problem assessment would be accurate and, even more important, acceptable.

To make the step of problem identification even more valid, we could have chosen to involve the community directly. By surveying a randomly chosen sample of our city's residents or by seeking opinions through an advertisement in the local newspaper, we could have been more certain that we were identifying a "real" community need.

When undertaking such a group process, a number of specific techniques can be used. We held informal, unstructured brainstorming sessions over coffee and cookies. Other group techniques, with names such as nominal group technique, Delphi process, and Ringi, are more structured and sophisticated (Horowitz & Gallagher, 1987). All of these methods could be described as qualitative.

Quantitative methods for identifying community needs exist as well. A large amount of data collected routinely can be of use. Census data provide age and gender distribution, employment information, ethnic background, marital status, language spoken, and socioeconomic status. Vital statistics give valuable information on birth and death rates, as well as causes of death. Mandatory reporting of communicable diseases such as STDs, TB, and some of the childhood exanthems provides a great deal of data that may be useful, especially if you believe that your community shows an unusual rate or distribution of a certain disease.

Quantitative data can be collected by the researcher specifically for the purpose of identifying community health problems; however, this can be expensive and time-consuming. Freeman (1987) described a method for estimating population-based rates of disease by "piggybacking" data collection onto other, patient-based (and useful) practice activities. The example he used involved an attempt to obtain an estimate of tuberculosis (TB) prevalence in a community. The practice already was planning an audit of diabetic care; it was known that most diabetics had TB skin tests done; and it was assumed that the prevalence of TB in the diabetic group was the same as in the larger community. Thus, as part of the data that were being collected for another purpose and at no additional cost or effort, the prevalence of TB was found (or at least estimated). This method could be applied to numerous other conditions and circumstances as a simple way to estimate population-based rates of disease or risk factors.

Another method for identifying and quantifying community health problems is one that I will call *microepidemiology*. If *epidemiology* is the study of the distribution and determinants of diseases in populations, then *microepidemiology* is the study of their distribution and determinants in micropopulations or, as they are called here, communities. It uses the same principles and methods as population epidemiology, but the object of measurement is a defined and qualified clinical community. (This type of research has been the strength of many of the great British GP researchers [Fry, 1988].) The results of a microepidemiological study can be of use in two ways. First, they must be of use to the community being studied. Second, they *may* be generalizable to other communities. An example will illustrate this.

In the community of "people in the Barrie area with STDs," we studied the prevalence of hepatitis B surface antigen positivity and found it to be much lower than other studies from large urban centers had reported (Morris et al., 1992). Because of this information, we decided *not* to screen routinely for hepatitis B in our STD clinic, a decision with obvious financial impact. As for the further use of these data, we believed that our results and conclusions were generalizable *to other similar communities* (small Canadian cities) (Morris et al., 1992).

This double impact of microepidemiology, first on the group being studied and then on other groups or populations, applies to all other types of community-based research as well. Because the research is being done *in, for,* and *by* the community, there must be a benefit to the community. Generalizability is a frequent, though not inevitable, bonus.

A potential problem arises if the needs as assessed by the community differ from the perception of the researcher. This problem can easily happen because of different belief systems, different knowledge, or vested interests on one side or the other. If negotiation does not lead to a compromise, then a practical solution (especially in the early stages of a collaboration) would be for the researcher to bend and agree to the community suggestion. If this is not done and the researcher imposes an agenda, the chances of further productive cooperation will be very slim.

RESPONDING TO COMMUNITY NEEDS

This is the third major step in the COPC paradigm. The community has been defined, and its needs (health problems) have been defined. What now? How do you respond to those needs?

How community needs are met depends on the problems that have been identified. Some problems will lend themselves to responses that are based in the practice. For instance, if undertreatment of hypertension is a problem and accessibility for follow-up is an obstacle, then a simple change in office hours may be part of the solution. If lower income families are unable to get to the office for care, then establishing an outreach office closer to them could help. If the physical layout of the office is a problem (for instance, physically handicapped patients cannot get their wheelchairs through doorways), then renovations will be necessary. If only a low proportion of elderly patients in the practice are being vaccinated against influenza on a yearly basis, then some type of reminder system will be needed (Rosser, 1987), whether this be during office visits for other reasons or by telephone or letter. In all of these examples, the response to important health problems involves a change within the physician's office.

Some community needs may require a response outside a single office. Recruitment of a new specialist or purchase of a new piece of investigative or therapeutic equipment might be the appropriate response to certain identified problems. These types of problems and responses usually are identified by physicians, rather than by the community as a whole. Other responses, however, will require the involvement of the whole community. For example, the program that we developed to deal with the problem of bicycle-related head injuries (and a bicycle helmet use rate of 5%) was planned by the same group that had identified this as a problem. The plan involved activities of all groups' participants, each in their own areas of expertise, coordinated by a steering group. Teachers organized school programs, service clubs hosted bicycle safety rodeos, physicians lobbied for mandatory legislation and promoted a reduced rate purchase scheme, retailers offered special discounts, displays were set up in local shopping malls, and extensive publicity accompanied everything. The benefits of widespread community involvement were apparent to all of us. The work load was shared, enthusiasm was kept high, and the issue was seen as a *community* problem, rather than as a crusade of one individual or group. And because the community "owned" the problem, impact was high.

This principle of sharing the work load applies equally to office- or practice-based community research. Nurses will have different (and equally valid) viewpoints on the nature of problems and solutions. Receptionists are *more* likely than the physician to hear about scheduling errors and other logistical problems. A practice that is large enough to have the services of a health educator has a valuable resource, who must be involved in all steps of the COPC process. By drawing on the abilities of all team members, the likelihood of success will be increased.

EVALUATING THE CHANGES

The fourth and final component of the response to community needs is to evaluate or monitor the program, also known as *program evaluation* or *quality assessment*. Whichever term is used, the principles remain the same. The first principle is simply that monitoring must be done. Second, monitoring should look, preferably, at the whole population at risk, not just at those involved in the program (in our bicycle helmet work, we counted the proportion of children wearing helmets in city parks and on randomly chosen streets, *not* just those outside bicycle shops or near schools whose teachers were involved in the program). And third, it must be sufficiently accurate to prove that the intervention program is truly doing what is desired (Nutting, 1987).

The community must not be viewed just as a laboratory in which we do our research (Seifert, 1982). It can and should be a source of ideas, with its members involved in setting the research agenda and determining priorities from beginning to end, including collaborative publication.

Community research is not just research *in* the community, but research *with, by,* and *for* the community.

COPC: A Practical Example From Israel

The practice of family medicine has three dimensions: care of the individual, care of the family, and care of the community. The last can present a major challenge, as it involves a change from the established focus of individual and family care.

In Israel, vocational training in family medicine has been promoted for the last 15 years by Kupat Holim, the health care organization responsible for the majority of primary health care delivery in the country. Kupat Holim community clinics exist in virtually every neighborhood in Israel, where they serve defined denominator populations.

The clinics have been characterized by long queues, poorly organized records, and lack of coordination of services. Complicating these problems has been the existence of an independent parallel service run by the Ministry of Health, providing primary care services to pregnant women and children. In addition, primary care services within Kupat Holim clinics have included separate services for women and children by primary care gynecologists and pediatricians. The primary care practitioners in the community clinics have been perceived to be principally "traffic agents" with inferior professional status and a poor image in the community.

The development of family medicine as a specialized discipline in Israel was motivated by these problems, as well as by the escalating costs of secondary and tertiary care. The existence of a defined denominator population has facilitated changes in the clinics and has enabled the development of a modified form of COPC, *community-oriented family medicine*. This approach is exemplified by the Rommema Clinic in Haifa, an urban teaching clinic with a denominator population of 6,200.

This clinic had been characterized by the stigma of Kupat Holim clinics in general. The change to a community-oriented family medicine approach involved four key steps:

1. *Introduction of an appointment system*, allowing for more effective control of services and resources, including the provision of community programs and after-hours services
2. *A team approach* that included medical secretaries, receptionists, nurses, and other health professionals, such as social workers
3. *Computerized problem-oriented medical records*
4. *Community involvement* in introducing changes

Needs were defined on the basis of community input and the characteristics of the denominator practice population, as well as epidemiological data on the Israeli population in general. As a first priority, three community programs were developed. The first was a women's health program, directed toward women aged 20 to 44, who constituted 40% of the practice population. This program included screening for cancer of the breast and cervix, organized in specific sessions. Many women presented with gynecological complaints and possible pathology that had not been identified prior to this program. The second program focused on hypertension and involved a door-to-door survey carried out by students, with measurement of blood pressure on all patients older than 10 years (Rennert, Strulov, Almagor, & Tamir, 1992). The third program was directed toward the elderly—a rapidly expanding part of the practice—and included a group of people who were frequent users of clinic services.

An evaluation of this program, conducted by the Department of Family and Community Health of Technion Medical School in Haifa, found improved patient satisfaction with the changed clinic services. It found an increased performance of breast self-examination; however, it also found a *lack* of screening for hypertension in this population.

In conclusion, community-oriented primary care is an achievable goal where programs are directed toward a defined population. Community involvement is a precondition to success. In Israel the introduction of this approach has been limited by a modest supply of qualified family physicians and by the need for structural changes in the existing primary health care system.

Note

1. Rhe Rummema Experience is funded by the Neeman Insitiute, Technion Hifa, and Kupat Holim Central Office under the leadership of Professor L. Epstein.

References

Freeman, W. L. (1987). "Piggybacking": The selective use of tracer-conditions from patient-based data to obtain population-based information useful for COPC. In P. A. Nutting (Ed.), *Community-oriented primary care: From principle to practice* (pp. 179-186). Washington, DC: U.S. Department of Health and Human Services.

Fry, J. (1988). *General practice and primary health care.* London: Nuffield Provincial Hospitals Trust.

Galazka, S. S., & Zyzanski, S. (1987). How representative is your practice population of the community? In P. A. Nutting (Ed.), *Community-oriented primary care: From principle to practice* (pp. 83-89). Washington, DC: U.S. Department of Health and Human Services.

Hawk, D. L., & Calvert, J. F. (1987). The active patients in a clinical practice: The first step toward a definable community. In P. A. Nutting (Ed.), *Community-*

oriented primary care: From principle to practice (pp. 40-44). Washington, DC: U.S. Department of Health and Human Services.

Hogg, W. E. (1984). Definition of the catchment area for a small rural hospital near a large city. *Canadian Family Physician, 30,* 326-332.

Horowitz, C., & Gallagher, K. M. (1987). Group process techniques for COPC practice. In P. A. Nutting (Ed.), *Community-oriented primary care: From principle to practice* (pp. 174-178). Washington, DC: U.S. Department of Health and Human Services.

Morris, B. A. P., & Butler-Jones, D. A. (1991). The role of the physician as community advocate. *Canadian Medical Association Journal, 144,* 1316-1317.

Morris, B. A. P., Harason, P., & Butler-Jones, D. A. (1992). Seroprevalence of hepatitis B in a small urban STD clinic. *Canadian Journal of Public Health, 83,* 73-74.

Morris, B. A. P., & Trimble, N. E. (1991). Promotion of bicycle helmet use among school children: A randomized clinical trial. *Canadian Journal of Public Health, 82,* 92-94.

New Webster's Dictionary and Thesaurus of the English Language. (1991). New York: Lexicon.

Nutting, P. A. (Ed.). (1987). *Community-oriented primary care: From principle to practice* (HRSA Publication No. HRS-A-PE 86-1). Washington, DC: U.S. Department of Health and Human Services.

Rennert, M., Strulov, A., Almagor, G., & Tamir, A. (1992). Hypertension and its implication to the family medicine team. *Harefuah, 122*(12), 757-759, 820.

Rosser, W. W. (1987). Strategies for clinical prevention in COPC. In P. A. Nutting (Ed.), *Community-oriented primary care: From principle to practice* (pp. 264-271). Washington, DC: U.S. Department of Health and Human Services.

Seifert, M. F. (1982). Research in family practice: A blueprint for the eighties. *Family Practice Research Journal, 1*(4), 211-223.

PART III

Collaborations

In Chapter 2, Dr. Herbert identified collaboration as one of the key elements required for quality research. Although individuals working alone can undertake useful research, the complexity of primary care lends itself to collaborative work. In Part III of this book we offer reflections on five collaborative arrangements.

In Chapter 9, Dr. Sangster and Ms. Gerace show how a physician and a nurse who practice collaboratively can both benefit from research done together in the practice. For many studies, however, the required sample sizes are larger than can be obtained in a single practice. This idea leads naturally to Chapter 10, in which Dr. Hickner discusses the strengths, weaknesses, and organization of successful networks of physicians doing collaborative research.

Collaboration in research between primary care physicians and the pharmaceutical industry has, in the past, been less than ideal. Dr. Hilditch, in Chapter 11, points out positive developments that have the potential to benefit the industry, family physicians, and patients. These developments are in the areas of postmarketing drug surveillance and quality of life studies.

In the last two chapters of Part III, attention turns to the academic setting. In Chapter 12, Dr. Macaulay looks at the benefits and risks of university-community collaboration from both sides. In Chapter 13, Drs. Brown and McWilliam identify the benefits and challenges of different disciplines working together on the same project.

Because of different paradigms and methodologies, consultation and cooperation are more common than true collaboration.

The one theme running through all five chapters is the necessity for mutual understanding, respect, and communication for effective collaboration.

9 Practice-Based Nurse/Physician Collaborative Research

JOHN F. SANGSTER
TOULA M. GERACE

Introduction

The family practice setting is an ideal environment in which the nurse and physician can establish a collaborative practice—that is, the provision of primary health care services to a defined and shared patient population. In the authors' opinion, this constitutes the basis for collaborative research as well. In this chapter we present a model of nurse/physician collaborative research based on the concept of *collaborative practice*.

The Case for Research Based in a Single Practice

Our concept of practice-based research is to view the practice as the laboratory, and the patients, or practice population, as the subjects of study. In primary health care, with its breadth and scope, researchable questions are endless; in addition, interventions by health care providers can be observed for both acceptability and effectiveness.

For practitioners who want to get involved in research, it is equally important to consider the value of conducting research *in one's own practice*. Doing so enables one to challenge conventional wisdom, to reconsider accepted ideas and actions, and to have the personal satisfaction of exploring one's curiosity about the events of daily practice (Geyman, 1978; McWhinney, 1966). Furthermore the experience gained can lead to new skills in record keeping and documentation, and by reviewing the literature on topics of interest, additional knowledge is acquired. In sum, the opportunity for self-improvement from being involved in the research process may well turn out to be one of the most important forms of continuing medical education.

Those involved in research may come to enjoy a new level of professional stimulation, both from the intellectual challenge and from the opportunities to share new information with like-minded colleagues. Gaining new insight into a specific problem that can be applied immediately to the practice population can be an extremely rewarding experience. The old concept of research only occurring at the molecular or bench level needs to be refocused to the pragmatic realities of daily practice: This adjustment will happen only when clinicians recognize the potential of practice-based research and envision their practice populations as "laboratories" for clinical research.

Most authorities on research stress the importance of conducting it in areas that have personal meaning or interest to the individual. It is this personal interest that will sustain the investigators to see projects through to their conclusion. It is equally important that the question selected for study be "doable"—that is, able to be accommodated comfortably within the current practice structure and answerable. Research that can be done while one is working in a day-to-day routine will have a greater likelihood of being completed and certainly can provide an added interest or incentive to daily practice. It has been stated that the ideal research study would be so integrated into the practice that only an experienced observer could tell that it was in progress. This type of union between clinical care and research has been described as an art and is believed to be essential for a productive research career in the practice setting (Berg, Gordon, & Cherkin, 1986).

Review of the historical medical literature provides examples of well-known clinician/researchers who have conducted practice-based research that subsequently has been shown to have had a major impact on medical practice. Pickles (1930, 1939) determined the incubation period and communicability of infectious hepatitis through simple record keeping, his knowledge of individuals in the community, and observing the natural history of the disease.

Spitzer (1977) identified that family practitioners have a distinct perspective on health care and have an obligation to study human beings in noninstitutionalized populations over long periods of time. They have the unique opportunity to observe transitions from health to disease and back to health again, along with many of the concurrent and contributing phenomena such as family issues, employment, housing, and exposure to risk factors. Similarly White (1976) noted the need to describe ambulatory care from the point of view of both providers and consumers, and the need for development of new techniques of data collection and analysis. He believed the focus might be on the personal, situational, and environmental factors associated with the onset of illness. Smith (1991) emphasized the ability of the practice-based investigator to observe patients longitudinally over time, a necessity for many research questions. He proposed that subjects in these types of studies are more representative of the general population than are those in studies originating in tertiary care settings and noted that primary-care practitioners are in a better position to study common health problems, as well as the delivery of health care. In sum, it is quite possible to envision the relevance and usefulness of practice-based research, as applied research, with an emphasis on improving practical decisions of patient care and health care delivery.

Dr. John Bain, professor of family medicine in Edinburgh, has used the phrase "small r research" to describe the feasibility of doing research projects in the practice setting (J. Bain, personal communication, October, 1991). Many of the results from "small r" studies can serve as excellent pilot projects for more major studies, which then can be developed further by full-time research teams into "big R" projects. Practitioners must be convinced of the importance of these small studies and conduct them, rather than hold back their curiosity because they think they do not have the time, experience, or skills to conduct larger ones. This is not to say that once an individual has experienced some success in completing small projects that he or she cannot consider larger and more complex ones, depending on interest and on cultivation of new and expanded research skills.

One of the criticisms leveled at single-practice-based research is the inherent limitation on sample size: Results obtained cannot be applied to the general population because of the potential bias associated with nonrepresentative small samples. Development of research networks for data collection has been one attempt to resolve this issue, launching the practitioner into a larger research network. However, not all physicians will believe they have the time or energy for this involvement and may end up discontinuing their research activity altogether. Freer (1987) said that the value of single-practice-based studies has not been fully appreciated and suggested that if more practices were encouraged rather than discouraged from doing small-scale studies, the combined power of the results might be much greater than we think. That is, consistent results from repeated small studies in different practices might be sufficient evidence for results to be generalized and could avoid the need for larger scale investigations. Such projects would be better directed toward those research areas where conflicting results have been found. Both "small r" and "big R" research projects are important to family practice and have a role to play in the future development of the discipline.

Despite all of the positive reasons for carrying out within-practice research, many practitioners find it difficult to do. The busy practitioner has many demands on his or her limited time and energy. Collaboration within the practice is one method of overcoming these difficulties. Our discussion focuses on nurse/physician collaboration in practice-based research.

Nurse/Physician Collaboration

Collaboration, simply defined, means working together to meet mutual goals. On the surface, this concept seems to be understood easily, yet when put in the framework of nurse/physician collaboration, it becomes more complex.

Nurses and physicians have worked together for many years, traditionally in a hierarchical fashion, with the physician holding the authoritative role of patient care manager and the nurse playing the deferential role of carrying out the physician's orders. Stein (1967) characterized this hierarchical relationship as the "doctor-nurse game," describing it as having rules, agreed to by both parties, that maintained the hierarchy. The cardinal rule of the game was that open disagreement had to be avoided at all costs. In 1990, Stein, Watts, and Howell reviewed the status of this game and determined that although it continues to be played in many places, it has been affected by a number of social changes forcing its modification toward a *collegial,* rather than a hierarchical, interaction. Such changes include a heightened public awareness of health and illness, the women's movement, and higher education of nurses.

The foundation of a true collegial relationship is mutual trust and respect, demanding open, honest, assertive communication shared laterally by both nurses and physicians. Several demonstration projects in the United States have featured a collaborative model of nurse/physician interaction characterized by such relationships. Participants in these projects have reported increased work satisfaction, a climate of confidence and trust, and positive responses from patients to the care they have received (Alt-White, Charns, & Strayer, 1983; Devereux, 1981a; Koerner, Cohen, & Armstrong, 1985).

Collaboration between nurses and physicians represents an interdependence between the two professions. Although each discipline has unique roles and philosophies, they share the common goals of preservation and restoration of health, as well as a number of skill sets, knowledge areas, and functions. Weiss and Davis (1985) defined *collaboration* in this case as the interactions between nurse and physician that enable the knowledge and skills of each to synergistically influence patient care. Problems associated with health and illness today tend to be so complex that it is unrealistic to think that one professional can manage them all completely. Together, nurses and physicians can provide a more comprehensive "package" of health care.

Collaborative Practice

Collaborative practice (also referred to as *associated* or *joint practice*) can develop from the collegial relationship, given the proper setting. In such an arrangement, the physician and the nurse mutually share responsibility for care of a specific population of patients (Elpern, Rodts, DeWald, & West, 1983). Descriptors used to explain the collaborative practice relationship include coequality, shared clients, interdependence, collegiality, shared accountability, cooperativeness, and joint decision making (McLain, 1988). Ames and Perrin (1980) emphasized that shared problem solving distinguishes collaborative practice from parallel practice, in which nurses and physicians work alongside each other in defined, independent paths.

Devereux (1981b) identified three essential components of collaborative practice: communication, competence, and accountability.

Communication is crucial not only to the planning and evaluation of patient care but also to interprofessional role perception. Brown (1974), in chronicling her involvement in the formation of a joint practice, found that development of collegial relations required time and trust to overcome basic professional differences. Traditional hierarchical attitudes initially interfered with the development of her role as an associate of the physicians with whom she was constructing the practice. Essential to change, both for her and for them, was communication regarding professional philosophies.

Competence is requisite to the establishment of mutual trust. Health professionals working together must have confidence in each other's knowledge and clinical skills in order to share and accept patient care decisions made by either of them.

Accountability implies the ability to assume responsibility for one's own clinical practice, taking ownership for one's decisions and actions (Puta, 1989).

Collaborative practice also can be compared to successful team functioning, wherein a team consists of two or more individuals. Larson and LaFasto (1989) stressed that a *collaborative climate* is the essence of teams. This climate is defined as the extent to which members communicate openly, disclose problems, share information, help each other overcome obstacles, and discover ways of effective problem solving. In their examination of effectively functioning teams, "working well together" was consistently described as a significant characteristic, with trust identified as the essential ingredient. A climate that included the four elements of honesty, openness, consistency, and mutual respect facilitated the development of trusting relationships.

Table 9.1 Relating Collaborative Practice to Maslow's Hierarchy of Needs

Self-actualization	Collaborative practice
Self-esteem	Nurse/physician collaboration
	Commitment to practice
	Accountability
Belonging	Collegial relationship
	Shared care
	Team
Safety and security	Honesty
	Trust
	Respect
	Competence
Basic needs	Communication

Rakel (1977) outlined criteria for effective teamwork:

1. Care of a defined group of patients is a shared responsibility; team members take care of the same patients.
2. Team members share common goals for patients and agree on how to reach these objectives.
3. Tasks are assigned to appropriate team members, and each recognizes, respects, and accepts the others' roles and responsibilities.
4. A communication mechanism is developed so that all can contribute and share the information essential for effective patient care.

The development of collaborative practice can be compared to Maslow's (1970) hierarchy of needs, more basic needs being prerequisite to the attainment of higher needs and, ultimately, "self-actualization." At the foundation is communication, analogous to basic needs, which takes precedence over all other levels. Collaborative practice, analogous to self-actualization, is the integration, achievement, and enactment of all lower levels. A comparison is shown in Table 9.1.

COLLABORATIVE FAMILY PRACTICE

Family practice can be viewed as a shared care environment in which each professional can perform clinically either independently or interdependently. Some overlapping areas of expertise, common to both nurse and physician, are highly interrelated; some areas are unique to each. As co-practitioners in a primary care setting, the nurse and physician, as a team, are committed to providing care to a defined and shared practice population. Aradine and Pridham (1973) stressed that co-practicing does not imply that both physician and nurse must see each patient at every visit or see each patient together. It does mean, however, that they establish a relationship with the patient and work together in a way that meets both of their needs and maintains their availability, responsibility, and relationship to the patient and family. Essential to establishing this relationship is obvious, open communication and commitment between them, and by each of them to the patient and to the practice. Without these, trust cannot develop, and each professional will be viewed as an individual practitioner, rather than as a co-practitioner.

COLLABORATIVE PRACTICE-BASED RESEARCH

Many of the principles of interprofessional collaboration apply to collaborative research as well. The fundamental difference is that the focus of attention changes from clinical practice alone to the question posed and how it will affect both provider and patient.

Research carried out in the practice setting can be conducted successfully by using a collaborative model only if all members of the team share a basic interest in doing the study. This is a cardinal tenet: If mutual interest does not exist, the research endeavor will be independent, rather than shared. Simply defined, *research* is organized curiosity. Asking the question is the first and most time-consuming step in the process; co-practitioners in collaborative practice who are motivated to do research are likelier to complete this step more productively and in a shorter period of time. They already have established open communication and, on the basis of their commitment to the practice, can determine what questions are relevant to them and to the population of patients they share.

Essential components of collaborative research include contribution, communication, commitment, and credit.

Contribution

A question that is explored by both the nurse and physician will have greater depth than one posed by either of them alone. Along with their common professional areas of knowledge, expertise, and experience, each contributes unique insights, thereby resulting in a much broader perspective of the question.

Research knowledge and experience may differ as well. The more seasoned researcher will make a greater contribution, giving the novice researcher an opportunity to learn more about the process through collaboration.

Communication

Like collaborative practice, collaborative research requires open, honest, and assertive communication. Between co-practitioners, a shift from communicating about clinical practice to communicating about the research process may threaten established patterns. If one member of the nurse/physician dyad feels unsure about his or her role in the research, communication may be affected adversely. It is imperative that this potentiality be addressed before research begins.

Commitment

For co-practitioners, commitment to a research question should come easily. Just as they are committed to the practice they share, they will be committed to the question because it will be related to the practice. Other types of commitment, however, such as time, work load, and finances, may not come so easily and will need to be negotiated.

Although one of the hallmarks of practice-based research is its incorporation into the daily routine, not enough time will be available for the entire process. Time outside of the regular work schedule must be devoted to the research undertaking; this may mean anything from 1 to 5 hours a week, depending on the stage of the project. Blocks of time, at least 2 hours per week, must be committed for reading, consulting, and thinking about the questions to be asked. If both researchers are willing to make this level of commitment, then the process can be maintained.

One of the major advantages of collaborative research is being able to share the work load. This sharing may mean equal distribution of the literature to be reviewed, equal participation in data collection, and equal contribution to writing the paper.

Collaboration enhances motivation: When the energy of one researcher wanes, the other is there to bolster it.

Finally every research project will differ in financial cost. The researchers may have to bear the burden of such cost and must be committed to sharing this equally.

Credit

Rules of authorship are sometimes difficult to apply to the nurse/physician collaborative research team. Stevens (1986), in reviewing criteria for authorship, noted that in the disciplines of medicine, pharmacy, and social work, it is agreed that the person writing the manuscript be the senior author, whereas in nursing and dentistry, senior authorship goes to the individual who assumed responsibility for designing the project. The American Psychological Association (1983) takes the position that the name of the principal contributor should appear first, with subsequent names in order of decreasing contribution.

When both the nurse and the physician are equal contributors, how do they decide about first authorship? They should discuss this at the initiation of the study and make a clear decision early on in order to avoid conflict about this potentially sensitive issue. The decision can be made in a number of ways: flipping a coin, taking turns from one publication to the next, or determining who needs publication credit at that particular time. Whatever method is used, it is imperative that both participants communicate and come to a mutually satisfactory decision.

EXAMPLES OF COLLABORATIVE RESEARCH

Improving Influenza Immunization Rates

Until recently, practitioners provided care primarily to those who attended the practice, with little thought to nonattending patients. This approach leads to gaps in the provision of preventive care. To remedy this deficiency, the concept of the practice as a population at risk, with all members deserving attention, has been championed (Nutting, 1987; Stott, 1987). In this model, a practice assumes responsibility for ensuring that the preventive care of all of its members is up to date.

To implement this model in our own practice, we undertook a research project to improve influenza vaccination for the elderly (Gerace & Sangster, 1988).

Immunization is a particularly important part of primary care for both physicians and nurses. They are in an ideal situation to actively identify and immunize patients of various age groups who are at risk. Although immunization is a sound preventive care strategy, influenza immunization rates continue to be less than acceptable, possibly a failure of health care providers to adequately offer the vaccine. It was apparent to us that when we began to examine our own practice pattern with respect to influenza immunization, it was inadequate, with only 17% of the elderly practice population being immunized annually. We agreed that an active attempt needed to be made to improve this rate substantially. We decided to undertake a study to compare the influence of two methods of outreach, over a 2-year period, on the rate of influenza immunization in the practice. We recognized that if the maximum number of at-risk elderly patients were to be offered immunization over the 2-month recommended time frame for administering influenza vaccine, all team members would need to be involved actively in identifying patients. Consequently both the physician and the nurse encouraged each other to offer influenza vaccine to elderly patients seen for any reason during the months of October and November in 1985 and 1986.

Furthermore, in November 1985, a letter was mailed to patients who had not been immunized by October 31. It informed them of the rationale for immunization, the potential side effects of the vaccine, and the availability and advisability of receiving it. The letter, which was signed personally by both the physician and the nurse, requested patients to contact the office if they wanted the vaccination. No follow-up was made of patients who did not respond to the letter.

In November 1986, patients who had not been immunized by October 31 were telephoned by the nurse to determine whether they were familiar with the vaccine. If appropriate, they were informed of the rationale for immunization, the potential side effects of the vaccine, and the availability and advisability of receiving it. Immunization rates were calculated and compared for both letter and telephone contact methods of outreach.

Clearly the outreach strategies were effective. The base immunization rate of 17% increased to 57.3% in 1985 and 65.6% in 1986. At first glance it would appear that the telephone outreach was the more successful one. In truth, it only resulted in an additional 16% of patients being immunized, while the letter outreach resulted in the immunization of a further 28.6% of patients. Perhaps the most significant factor in the enhanced immunization rates was the improvement in offering vaccine to patients.

In this study it was imperative that active, ongoing *communication* take place, not only regarding the interest in and perceived importance of the question of study but also in offering vaccine to patients. We consistently reminded each other of the time frame for vaccination, identified patients at risk to each other, and reviewed the progress of our enhanced awareness of influenza vaccination to each other.

The *contributions* of the physician and the nurse differed somewhat, with the physician and the nurse both taking responsibility for producing and signing the outreach letters and the nurse alone making the outreach by telephone.

The *commitment* to the project was shared equally with respect to the identification of patients at risk, meeting regularly to review our progress, and sharing the work of reviewing literature, planning the outreach strategies, analyzing our final data, and writing it up for publication. Financial cost of mailing the outreach letters was absorbed by the practice.

Because the bulk of the actual outreach was carried out by the nurse, as well as the actual physical act of immunizing patients, we thought that credit of first authorship for the final paper most appropriately went to the nurse (Gerace & Sangster, 1988).

Testing for Hearing Loss

Another research question was generated by the introduction of a new technology into the practice: the Welch Allyn audioscope (Sangster, Gerace, & Seewald, 1991). Although we recognized that hearing loss was a significant problem for the elderly, screening for such loss was not something we routinely did in the practice. After reviewing the literature, we found that not only was the audioscope recommended for screening the elderly for hearing loss but a simple questionnaire known as the Hearing Handicap

Inventory for the Elderly (HHIE) was as well. However, both forms of screening had been used very little in the primary care family practice setting. We decided to assess the effectiveness of both screening tools in the practice in order to determine whether the audioscope alone, the HHIE alone, or the audioscope in conjunction with the HHIE would best identify those individuals with a hearing impairment. The objectives were (a) to identify individuals with a hearing impairment, (b) to compare the primary screening with a "gold standard" audiogram, and then (c) to recommend a hearing aid if necessary. We found the prevalence of hearing loss was 30% among the elderly in the practice. When compared to the "gold standard" audiological assessment, the audioscope was found to be an effective method of screening on its own in the primary care family practice setting.

In this study, *communication* about the importance of the problem of hearing loss among the elderly, as well as the testing of a new technology introduced into the practice, was essential. We agreed that, from both a medical and a nursing perspective, the identification of elderly patients with hearing loss was important. As co-practitioners, we agreed it was equally important to evaluate the introduction of new technology into our practice.

The *contributions* of the physician and the nurse differed somewhat in this study as well. Although both the physician and the nurse identified patients who were invited to participate in the study, the nurse administered the questionnaire, whereas the physician physically examined the ears of the participants and tested their hearing with the audioscope.

The *commitment* to this project again was shared equally with respect to the identification of potential participants, meeting regularly to review our progress, and sharing the work of reviewing the literature, interpreting the data analysis, and writing the paper for publication. There was no financial cost to the practice.

Because the physician was responsible for examining and testing hearing with the audioscope, we thought that credit of first authorship most appropriately went to the physician (Sangster et al., 1991).

Subsequent to this "small r" pilot study in our own practice, funding for a similar "big R" study was obtained and carried out among nine community family practices in London, Ontario.

One of the most exciting aspects of practice-based research is to be able to apply the impact of the results of a project within the practice setting almost as soon as it is known. It takes approximately another 12 months for results to be disseminated in the literature, but by then the cycle of starting on the next project and collecting data can already be well under way. Thus a constant sequence of formulating a question, reviewing the literature, collecting data on the practice population, analyzing these data, presenting the results, and writing them up for publication can be kept in motion by a few hours per week. The sense of accomplishment that comes from following this process can provide a great sense of personal satisfaction, a sense of improving patient care within the practice, an opportunity to share this experience with others, and a sense of making a contribution to the literature. This experience becomes intrinsically rewarding and can help maintain a high level of interest in the day-to-day practice for both the physician and the nurse.

References

Alt-White, A. C., Charns, M., & Strayer, R. (1983). Personal, organizational, and managerial factors related to nurse-physician collaboration. *Nursing Administration Quarterly, 8*, 8-18.

American Psychological Association. (1983). *Publication manual of the American Psychological Association* (3rd ed.). Washington, DC: Author.

Ames, A., & Perrin, J. M. (1980). Collaborative practice: The joining of two professions. *Journal of the Tennessee Medical Association, 73*(8), 557-560.

Aradine, C. R., & Pridham, K. F. (1973). Model for collaboration. *Nursing Outlook, 21*(10), 655-657.

Berg, A. O., Gordon, M. J., & Cherkin, D. C. (1986). *Practice-based research in family medicine.* Kansas City, KS: American Academy of Family Physicians.

Brown, K. C. (1974). The nurse practitioner in a private group practice. *Nursing Outlook, 22*(2), 108-113.

Devereux, P. M. (1981a). Does joint practice work? *Journal of Nursing Administration, 11*(6), 39-43.

Devereux, P. M. (1981b). Essential elements of nurse-physician collaboration. *Journal of Nursing Administration, 11*(5), 19-23.

Elpern, E. H., Rodts, M. F., DeWald, R. L., & West, J. W. (1983). Associated practice: A case for professional collaboration. *Journal of Nursing Administration, 13*(11), 27-31.

Freer, C. B. (1987). The case for small practice-based studies. *Family Practice Research Journal, 6*(3), 120-122.

Gerace, T. M., & Sangster, J. F. (1988). Influenza vaccination: A comparison of two outreach strategies. *Family Medicine, 20*(1), 43-45.

Geyman, J. P. (1978). On the developing research base in family practice. *Journal of Family Practice, 7*(1), 51-52.

Koerner, B. L., Cohen, J. R., & Armstrong, D. M. (1985). Collaborative practice and patient satisfaction: Impact and selected outcomes. *Evaluation and the Health Professions, 8*(3), 299-321.

Larson, C. E., & LaFasto, F. M. J. (1989). *Teamwork: What must go right/What can go wrong.* Newbury Park, CA: Sage.

Maslow, A. H. (1970). *Motivation and personality.* New York: Harper & Row.

McLain, B. R. (1988). Collaborative practice: The nurse practitioner's role in its success or failure. *Nurse Practitioner, 13*(5), 31-38.

McWhinney, I. R. (1966). General practice as an academic discipline. *Lancet, 1,* 419.

Nutting, P. A. (1987). Population-based family practice: The next challenge of primary care. *Journal of Family Practice, 24*(1), 83-88.

Pickles, W. (1930). Epidemic catarrhal jaundice: An outbreak in Yorkshire. *British Medical Journal, 1,* 944-946.

Pickles, W. (1939). *Epidemiology in country practice.* Bristol, UK: John Wright.

Puta, D. F. (1989). Nurse-physician collaboration toward quality. *Journal of Nursing Quality Assurance, 3*(2), 11-18.

Rakel, R. E. (1977). *Principles of family medicine.* Philadelphia: W. B. Saunders.

Sangster, J. F., Gerace, T. M., & Seewald, R. C. (1991). Hearing loss in elderly patients in a family practice. *Canadian Medical Association Journal, 144*(8), 981-984.

Smith, F. O. (1991). Practice-based research: Opportunities for the clinician. *Southern Medical Journal, 84*(4), 479-481.

Spitzer, W. O. (1977). The intellectual worthiness of family medicine. *Alpha Omega Alpha, 402,* 2.

Stein, L. I. (1967). The doctor-nurse game. *Archives of General Psychiatry, 16,* 699-703.

Stein, L. I., Watts, D. T., & Howell, T. (1990). The doctor-nurse game revisited. *New England Journal of Medicine, 322*(8), 546-549.

Stevens, K. R. (1986). Authorship: Yours, mine, or ours? *Image: Journal of Nursing Scholarship, 18*(4), 151-154.

Stott, N. C. (1987). Research in general practice: A rapidly changing scene. *Practitioners, 231,* 929-930.

Weiss, S. J., & Davis, H. P. (1985). Validity and reliability of the collaborative practice scales. *Nursing Research, 34,* 299-305.

White, K. L. (1976). Primary care research and the new epidemiology. *Journal of Family Practice, 3,* 579.

10 Practice-Based Network Research

JOHN HICKNER

Introduction

Compared with researchers in other medical disciplines, family practice researchers are underfunded, undertrained, and severely outnumbered. Yet high-quality, original research is necessary for the survival and growth of family medicine. Members of the discipline are beginning to live up to this challenge, in part, by using a tremendously powerful laboratory—their own offices. No other specialty has such ready access to millions of patients of all ages presenting with unfiltered complaints and illnesses. This untapped potential was recognized years ago by British general practice research pioneers Will Pickles (Pemberton, 1970) and John Fry (Fry, 1988) and more recently by Curtis Hames, a general practitioner from Georgia (Hames, 1992). Their work provides inspiration to aspiring family practice researchers today.

Family practice offices become even more powerful laboratories when networks of offices pool their patient data to yield large sample sizes in an efficient manner, giving results of greater generalizability. Research in these settings is called *practice-based network research*. The concept of doing research in this way is not new; multicenter studies have been funded by the National Institutes of Health for many years. Most notable are cancer treatment protocols and the large cardiovascular studies of hypertension, stroke, and acute myocardial infarction, for the most part consisting of randomized clinical trials to determine the effectiveness of drugs or other interventions. Another example of early work is the studies by a group of community pediatricians in Rochester, New York, on antibiotic prophylaxis for recurrent otitis media (Perrin et al., 1974). In family medicine circles, the Dutch Sentinel Stations, a network of general practices in The Netherlands, have reported continuously since 1970 and have investigated more than 60 topics (Green & Lutz, 1990).

What *is* new is the rapidly growing popularity of these networks as laboratories for family medicine investigators, not only in North America but also in Europe and Australia. An inventory of sentinel health information systems with general practitioners in Europe lists network activity in 12 countries. Of these, 7 networks in France, 5 in Great Britain, 5 in Spain, and 10 in The Netherlands gather data on a wide range of illnesses (Van Casteren, 1991).

I have divided this chapter into four sections. In the first part I discuss the reasons for this rapid growth in practice-based primary care research networks. In the second, third, and fourth sections I discuss the mechanics of establishing a network, some of the logistical issues important for successful studies, and some of the strengths and limitations, respectively. The information presented here draws heavily from two U.S. government reports published by the Agency for Health Care Policy and Research: Green and Lutz (1990) and Hickner (1991).

Reasons for the Popularity of Practice-Based Network Research

Perhaps a bit of autobiography will help illustrate the growing popularity of practice-based network research. After completing my family practice training at the Medical University of South Carolina in 1978, I took a job teaching and practicing at the very rural Upper Peninsula Campus of Michigan State University College of Human Medicine. Located 400 miles from the main medical school campus, this small program was designed to train medical students with a professed interest in rural medicine. Although my main duties were patient care and teaching, with the little time remaining I decided to satisfy my intellectual curiosity with some office research. After a few frustrating, nonproductive years, I learned the first secret of successful research for a busy clinician and teacher—collaboration. And not necessarily with Madame

Curie or James Watson—with a physician assistant and medical students, in my case! My interest in preventive medicine steered us to a project on fluoride supplementation for caries prevention and then to one on smoking cessation during pregnancy (Hickner, Westenberg, & Dittenbir, 1984; Messimer & Hickner, 1983). With the second project, we decided to go from descriptive studies to a clinical trial. With only 60 deliveries a year in our practice, a 20% smoking rate, and the need for at least 35 patients per group, we would have been enrolling patients for 6 years! Instead we recruited five other practices and completed enrollment in 6 months and the entire study in 15 months (Messimer, Hickner, & Henry, 1989).

This sketch illustrates two of the strongest attractions of practice-based network research: the opportunity to collaborate with others who have similar interests, and the need to recruit more patients than may be readily available in a single practice.

The issue of large numbers is one of the main reasons for the success of the Ambulatory Sentinel Practice Network (ASPN), a large binational research network in the United States and Canada. Founded as an offshoot of the North American Primary Care Research Group in 1980, ASPN undertakes studies that require large patient populations. For example, although headache is a common complaint in primary care, serious causes of headache such as subdural hematoma or brain tumor are not. How often are family doctors worried enough about serious pathology to order a computerized tomography (CT) brain scan for headache? To study this frequency, ASPN was able to amass 4,940 patient visits for headache in 14 months. Not surprisingly to family doctors, but contrary to most neurology texts, CT scans were ordered in only 3.0% of cases (Becker et al., 1987).

An even more compelling reason for the importance of practice-based research is the issue of generalizability. The classic work of White (White, Williams, & Greenberg, 1961) explains why family doctors feel uncomfortable with patient evaluation and management recommendations from university centers. White and his colleagues studied the frequency of illness in a general population and the filtering process that takes place before patients present for care at various levels of the health care system. In one month, 750 of 1,000 adults will have a medical complaint, and 250 will contact their doctors for care. Only 1, however, will be referred to a university center. A fraction of those referred will be entered into randomized clinical trials on which specialists will base their current recommendations for evaluation and treatment. Basing care on these referral patients will not work for the rural physician whose patients rarely travel farther than the nearest city. This patient population is different in many ways from the patients cared for in highly specialized, academic tertiary care centers. Family physicians recognize the conflict between what is written in standard texts and what they see in their own practices. Only by studying patients similar to his or her own will the primary care physician be able to provide optimal care. Network research allows this to happen.

I chose the rural illustration not only because of my rural background but also as another illustration of the problem of generalizability. Because most studies are done in urban medical centers drawing on urban populations, rural dwellers are tremendously underrepresented. I do not wish to push the rural argument to the absurd, because people are similar in most ways whether they live in the city or in the country. There are notable differences, nonetheless, and these differences can be appreciated only by studying them.

ASPN's collaborative study with the Centers for Disease Control and Prevention (CDC) about HIV seropositivity is illustrative. Because of ASPN's size and national distribution, the CDC has worked with this network to monitor the frequency of HIV seropositivity in a primary care population. Many of the ASPN practices are rural, and the HIV seropositivity rate appears much lower than average in many rural areas (unpublished ASPN data). Consistent with this observation, our rural research group, the Upper Peninsula Research Network, studied the prevalence of *Chlamydia trachomatis* infections in five family practice offices (Root, Hickner, & Nelson, 1991). We found a 4.6% prevalence, much less than in urban family planning clinics, but similar to a suburban family practice setting (Willard & Edman, 1989). These differences show that not only geographic location but also practice type determines the kind of patients seen.

Another point regarding generalizability concerns the idiosyncrasies of practice style. Each of us has a certain way of approaching problems and a certain personality that attracts certain patients. This uniqueness makes me wary of accepting the results of studies based in a single practice. For example, Solberg (Solberg, Maxwell, Kottke, Gepner, & Brekke, 1990) reported being able to decrease markedly the rate of smoking of patients in his practice by "gearing up" his entire office staff to promote cessation. Although I am a staunch antismoker, I am not certain that I have the personal zeal to do so well. Do I measure myself as a failure if I do less well? Do his results set the standard? I think not. (Though perhaps the ideal!) Studies of larger, more homogeneous groups of patients and doctors would allow me to put more stock in the findings.

I have one more issue about generalizability, this one concerning the patients who actually participate in a study, compared to those who are recruited. Large national, randomized trials filter many patients before arriving at the actual study population. For example, in the Systolic Hypertension in the Elderly Program (SHEP Cooperative Research Group, 1991), only 24% of those screened who were invited and met the initial enrollment criteria actually reported for the first study visit. The resulting samples may be very well described but are not very representative of common patients with the condition being studied. In our study of *C. trachomatis* infections, the refusal rate was only 2% among 593 eligible participants (Root et al., 1991).

A new generation of academic family physicians who have interest and training in research methods recognizes the potential of this type of collaboration and is creating a growing demand for the laboratories of practice-based network research. An informal survey in 1988 by the American Academy of Family Physicians of its state chapters listed 25 family practice research networks in the United States.

Yet another force driving network research is the refreshing interest in preventive medicine research. Determining the effectiveness of health education interventions and health screening requires epidemiologic methods and large sample sizes. A tremendous opportunity exists to study screening and prevention in family doctors' offices, which is where most preventive services originate. Even the United States government recently has recognized the value of studying patients in primary care settings. For example, the Agency for Health Care Policy and Research (AHCPR), established in 1990 by congressional mandate, includes a Division of Primary Care, which has an expressed interest in practice-based network research.

Here is a summary of the reasons behind the popularity of practice-based network research: The practice is the clinical laboratory of the family doctor. Much of family practice research, especially trials of prevention and screening, requires epidemiological methods with large patient populations. Issues of generalizability demand that family doctors study their own patient populations to provide the best care tailored to the diseases and needs of their patients. And finally, the academic family practice community is growing in number and sophistication.

Establishing a Network

Before "getting the faith" and rushing to establish a network, an investigator must decide whether more than one practice is indeed needed for a study. A single large group practice will suit many studies, and multipractice studies mean multiproblem studies when it comes to coordination, communication, and control of data quality. Even supposing your study requires more than one practice for success, establishing a formal network with all of the accompanying administrative maintenance is not a prerequisite. A group of practices can be brought together for a single study without any implication of a long-term relationship. Our clinical trial of smoking cessation took place in three family practice offices and three ob-gyn offices that had not collaborated previously or since. On the one hand, this approach has certain advantages: It is clean—get in and get out; it avoids overtaxing the practices; and it provides a fresh patient population that has not been "studied out." On the other hand, greater time and energy are necessary to train the doctors and staffs of offices unfamiliar with research protocols, and data quality may suffer initially.

After much soul-searching, you have decided that a network of practices with a more enduring commitment to research is to your liking. Good news! Establishing a research network is no longer pure guesswork; several groups have published information about their policies, procedures, and histories (Christoffel et al., 1988; Nelson et al., 1981). Directors of six primary care research networks pooled their collective wisdom at a workshop during a conference entitled Primary Care Research: Theory and Methods, sponsored by AHCPR in 1991 (Hickner, 1991). The following discussion draws heavily on their deliberations.

GETTING STARTED

Without a doubt, getting off the ground depends a good deal on the enthusiasm and commitment of at least one and ideally two or more individuals. Clearly identify and understand your expectations: Networks can be built around many different issues. Some examples: The Clinical Experience Network (1990) has been involved in drug-related trials. ASPN focuses on common problems seen in primary care that require large sample sizes to study and hopes for wide generalizability of results. NaReS (National Research System, of the College of Family Physicians of Canada) was formed in 1976 in response to the prospect of a swine flu epidemic (Lewis, 1989) and since then has taken on a wide variety of projects. The Wisconsin Research Network's (WReN) philosophy is to involve as many family doctors in Wisconsin as possible. The Upper Peninsula Research Network (UPRNet) is both a rural research network and a rural teaching network for medical students with primary care interests. A network could begin with an area focus such as prevention or screening.

Know *why* you want to conduct network research: If you have no personal compelling reason, maybe your time would be better spent in other research endeavors. You must determine who else cares about your project. Is it of interest only to an academic department, or does it have support among the community family doctors? Any successful primary care network must have strong support and significant input from the community practitioners, who must feel ownership of it. In both the Dartmouth COOP network in New England and in ASPN, forceful feedback from practitioners has caused major changes in policies, resulting in stronger networks. Empowering the practicing clinicians formally in the governing board of the network will pay major dividends.

The commitment of academic colleagues and community practitioners is not enough. Research costs money—not only to run the studies but also for administrative costs related to communication, travel, and secretarial staffing. According to Green and

Lutz (1990), "Buttressed with a strong spirit of volunteerism, approximately $50,000 per year for each of at least 3 years is sufficient to launch a network and determine its feasibility" (p. 126). Fifty thousand dollars is no small piece of change, but some of these costs can be absorbed by gaining a firm commitment from an existing administrative structure such as a family practice department, a state family practice chapter, or a foundation. Private foundation and government grants have been a source of start-up funds for several networks, including ASPN, COOP, WReN, and UPRNet.

A low-budget approach is certainly possible. The Michigan Research Network (MIRNET), established in 1984 by Drs. Doug McKeag and John Hickner of Michigan State University, began as a very loose association of six practices. With three medical schools in the state interested in participating, MIRNET eventually found a home in the Research Committee of the Michigan Academy of Family Physicians (MAFP). MAFP provides a part-time secretary at $1,400 per year, and each family practice department from the state's three medical schools contributes $1,000 per year for administrative support. This small funding base allows regular communication between the practices by monthly phone conferences, publication of a descriptive brochure, and start-up funds for small projects. Larger studies have been funded with project-specific grants from a variety of sources.

MIRNET is just one example of many administrative structures adopted by primary care research networks. Of the others mentioned here, ASPN is a totally independent organization, governed by a board of directors and incorporated as a not-for-profit organization in Virginia, though the central office is housed in the Department of Family Medicine at the University of Colorado Health Sciences Center (Green et al., 1984). WReN is part of the Wisconsin Institute of Family Medicine, the charitable arm of the Wisconsin Academy of Family Physicians, and its director is a faculty member of the Department of Family Medicine of the University of Wisconsin Medical School (Beasley et al., 1991). Pediatric Research in Office Settings (PROS) is sponsored and supported by the American Academy of Pediatrics. NaReS is sponsored by the College of Family Physicians of Canada. The Dartmouth COOP Project was governed originally by the faculty of Dartmouth's Department of Community Medicine and has since been restructured with a board composed of six community practitioners and one representative of the Department of Community and Family Medicine at Dartmouth. UPRNet is a project of the rural Upper Peninsula Campus of Michigan State University. In addition, many family practice departments across Canada and the United States have informal practice-based regional networks.

MAINTAINING THE NETWORK

By their nature, networks are spread out geographically, so daily contact is not possible. Regular communication is an essential survival tactic. Because correspondences to busy practitioners rapidly find their way to the circular file, communiques must be tied to specific objectives. Developing and maintaining a sense of identity with the network should be a major goal. Plaques, certificates, and newsletters help serve this purpose. Regular feedback of interim results and prompt reporting of final results to practitioners prior to publication are useful. Including practitioners in project development creates a sense of ownership and often keeps a project on target for the needs of family doctors. The importance of rewarding participation of doctors and their office staffs cannot be overemphasized. In busy family practice offices, a research study is just one more thing to do for an already overworked staff. Rewards may include recognition, money, thank-you notes, even a box of chocolates.

Unfortunately, goodwill does not pay the bills. All networks must grapple with funding issues. Ultimately, funded projects will fuel high activity, but some minimal infrastructure support is needed to carry the network through lean times. Eventually indirect cost reimbursement from grants can support the infrastructure, though this is unlikely in the early phases of development. For networks interested in drug trials, the pharmaceutical industry can be a source of support (see Chapter 11). (The Royal Academy of General Practitioners of New Zealand has capitalized on this source of funding in a major and constructive way.) All primary care research networks I am aware of have had to rely, in part, on an institutional parent for financial support.

Conducting Studies
in Practice-Based Networks

Now to the nitty-gritty. How does one actually run a practice-based network study? If the study happens to be a large NIH cancer or cardiac drug trial, the correct answer is "with lots of money, lots of research assistants, and lots of consultants." Truth is embedded in this facetious answer. Practice-based studies are not easy: They require enormous amounts of cooperation, coordination, and communication. All of the basic principles of sound scientific inquiry must be applied in a very uncontrolled laboratory setting—a basic scientist's nightmare. However, the real world of family doctors is their most legitimate laboratory. So study we must! Research in private doctors' offices poses unique obstacles, which I will discuss further in the concluding section. An entire textbook could be devoted to methodology of practice-based network studies; following are a few caveats from those who have tried it:

1. Allow the practitioners to give input at an early stage of project development. This is the only way to ensure their interest and keep the project on target.

2. The research project team should include at least one academic and one practicing doctor. The latter often comes up with excellent research ideas but lacks the time and expertise to carry a project through to completion.

3. Identify a member of each office staff to serve as the "practice coordinator" for studies. The coordinators stay close to the action and effectively monitor the study. This role usually is filled by an office nurse.

4. Take time to train the practicing physicians and office staffs. If they understand the study background and the methodology clearly, data quality will be enhanced.

5. Keep protocols as simple as possible (unless you can afford to hire research assistants to go into the practices to collect the data). If data collection instruments are simple and practical, the odds of accurate data recording are increased.

6. Do not overload the network with studies. (ASPN has used an effective card system for recording data on two or three studies simultaneously; however, each study gathers only a limited amount of information.)

7. A short, intense period of data gathering of 2 or 3 months works better than more prolonged reporting for most studies. "Reporting fatigue" has been noted by ASPN, with returns tapering off after a few months.

8. Longer studies can be successful when frequent communication with and feedback to the practitioners are promoted. Such studies should have less intense reporting needs; otherwise "reporting fatigue" sets in and data quality suffers.

9. Networks are uncontrolled laboratories. Incorporate data quality checks into the protocol whenever possible.

10. Providing regular feedback to the practitioners during the course of the study may enhance data quality.

Strengths and Limitations of Practice-Based Network Research

Green and Lutz (1990) listed several important advantages of practice-based research networks. First, networks have the potential to "access neglected phenomena of great importance to people" in primary care settings, producing results with wide generalizability. Second, there can be great efficiency because similar protocols and procedures can be applied to a number of studies with minimal retraining. (As mentioned above, with well-constructed data-gathering instruments, ASPN runs two or three studies simultaneously.) Third, large networks can study infrequent events in relatively short periods of time. Fourth, networks link academic expertise with community clinicians to produce new information of practical daily value to family doctors. This "town-gown" link is critical to the development and credibility of the specialty of family practice, whose practitioners have been criticized by their specialty colleagues for practicing unscientific, "seat-of-the-pants" medicine: It may encourage family doctors to practice better medicine and to maintain a critical attitude toward their own practice habits. Finally, as stated previously, family physicians' offices are the ultimate clinical laboratories for family medicine.

Holloway (1991) believes the value of practice-based research networks has been overstated. Although he agrees with their goals, he thinks they are expensive and cumbersome, and he states that there is no convincing evidence that ambulatory patients of residency- and university-affiliated clinics are different from ambulatory patients elsewhere. He agrees, however, that rural and international networks have unique potential to study variations in practice, as well as other comparative aspects.

Green and Lutz (1990) cogently summarized some of the limitations of networks, recognizing that inadequately developed theory and methods are major hurdles to overcome. For example, how does one best ensure data quality? Data collection and assessment must be accurate in the practices, with the appropriate data collected and collected completely, yet the best methods to ensure quality data from practices are not yet fully understood. The tremendous amount of communication and coordination might be perceived as a limitation, but it is one that can be overcome with sufficient time and attention. At times, the practitioners can be a weak link in the data collection process because of multiple competing demands in busy clinical settings. Intervention trials in practitioners' offices have major methodological challenges because they are time-consuming and also pose significant ethical dilemmas where the doctor feels the pull between caring for the patient and following the protocol. This dilemma, of course, is not unique to network research (Hellman & Hellman, 1991). And finally, funding network administrative costs will remain a stumbling block until established medical research funding agencies recognize the full potential of practice-based research networks to produce important findings for patient care.

References

Beasley, J. W., Cox, N. S., Livingston, B. T., Davis, J. E., McBride, P., Hankey, T. L., Shropshire, R., & Roberts, R. G. (1991). Development and operation of the Wisconsin Research Network. *Wisconsin Medical Journal, 90,* 531-537.

Becker, L. A., Iverson, D. C., Reed, F. M., Calonge, B. N., Miller, R. S., & Freeman, W. L. (1987). A study of headache in North American primary care: A report from the Ambulatory Sentinel Practice Network. *Journal of the Royal College of General Practitioners, 37,* 400-403.

Christoffel, K. K., Binns, H. J., Stockman III, J. A., McGuire, P., Poncher, J., Unti, S., Typlin, B., Lasin, G., & Seigel, W. (1988). Practice-based research: Opportunities and obstacles. *Pediatrics, 82,* 399-405.

Clinical Experience Network. (1990). A large-scale, office-based study evaluates the use of a new class of nonsedating antihistamines. *Journal of the American Board of Family Practice, 3,* 241-252.

Fry, J. (1988). *General practice and primary health care 1940s-1980s.* London, UK: Nuffield Provincial Hospitals Trust.

Green, L. A., & Lutz, L. (1990). Notions about networks: Primary care practices in pursuit of improved primary care. In J. Mayfield & M. L. Grady (Eds.), *Primary care research: An agenda for the 90s* (pp. 125-132). Rockville, MD: Agency for Health Care Policy and Research.

Green, L. A., Wood, M., Becker, L., Farley, E. S., Freeman, W. L., Froom, J., Hames, C., Niebauer, L. J., Rosser, W. W., & Seifert, M. (1984). The Ambulatory Sentinel Practice Network: Purpose, methods, and policies. *Journal of Family Practice, 18,* 275-280.

Hames, C. (1992). In the eyes of the beholder: A thirty-year odyssey of research in primary care. In M. Stewart, F. Tudiver, M. J. Bass, E. V. Dunn, & P. G. Norton (Eds.), *Tools for primary care research* (pp. 1-13). Newbury Park, CA: Sage.

Hellman, S., & Hellman, D. S. (1991). Of mice but not men: Problems of the randomized clinical trial. *New England Journal of Medicine, 324,* 1585-1589.

Hickner, J. (1991). Practice-based primary care research networks. In H. Hibbard, P. A. Nutting, & M. L. Grady (Eds.), *Primary care research: Theory and methods* (pp. 13-22). Rockville, MD: Agency for Health Care Policy and Research.

Hickner, J., Westenberg, C., & Dittenbir, M. (1984). Effect of pregnancy on smoking behavior: A baseline study. *Journal of Family Practice, 2,* 241-242.

Holloway, R. L. (1991). Networks and net worth: Practice-based data collection in family medicine. *Journal of Family Practice, 33,* 137-139.

Lewis, J. (1989). NaReS: Your research system. *Canadian Family Physician, 35,* 837-839.

Messimer, S., & Hickner, J. (1983). Oral fluoride supplementation: Improving practitioner compliance by using a protocol. *Journal of Family Practice, 7,* 567-576.

Messimer, S., Hickner, J., & Henry, R. (1989). A comparison of two antismoking interventions among pregnant women in eleven private primary care practices. *Journal of Family Practice, 3,* 283-288.

Nelson, E. C., Kirk, J. W., Bise, B. W., Chapman, R. J., Hale, F. A., Stamps, P. L., & Wasson, J. H. (1981). The Cooperative Information Project: Part 1: A sentinel practice network for service and research in primary care. *Journal of Family Practice, 13,* 641-649.

Pemberton, J. (1970). *Will Pickles of Wensleydale.* London, UK: Royal College of General Practitioners.

Perrin, J., Charney, E., MacWhinney, J. B. Jr., McInerny, T. K., Miller, R. L., & Nazarian, L. F. (1974). Sulfisoxazole as chemoprophylaxis for recurrent otitis media: A double-blind crossover study in pediatric practice. *New England Journal of Medicine, 291,* 664-667.

Root, D. T., Hickner, J. M., & Nelson, T. C. (1991). Prevalence and prediction of chlamydial cervical infection in a rural area: An UPRNet Project. *Journal of Family Practice, 4,* 369-374.

SHEP Cooperative Research Group. (1991). Prevention of stroke by antihypertensive drug treatment in older persons with isolated systolic hypertension: Final results of the Systolic Hypertension in the Elderly Program (SHEP). *Journal of the American Medical Association, 265,* 3255-3302.

Solberg, L. I., Maxwell, P. L., Kottke, T. E., Gepner, G. J., & Brekke, M. L. (1990). A systematic primary care office-based smoking cessation program. *Journal of Family Practice, 30*, 647-654.

Van Casteren, V. (1991). *Inventory of sentinel health information systems with GPs in the European Community.* Brussels: Institute of Hygiene and Epidemiology.

White, K. L., Williams, F., & Greenberg, B. G. (1961). The ecology of medical care. *New England Journal of Medicine, 265*(18), 885-889.

Willard, M. A., & Edman, R. L. (1989). Screening for genital *Chlamydia trachomatis* in female patients in a primary care setting. *Journal of Family Practice, 28*, 97-98.

11 Industry-Sponsored Research

JOHN R. HILDITCH

The contribution of the pharmaceutical industry to medical research funding is becoming increasingly important (Council on Scientific Affairs and Council on Ethical and Judicial Affairs, 1990; Ryten, 1991). During the years from 1981 to 1990, its contribution to biomedical research in Canadian universities increased from 2% to 8.3% of the total funding. The annual rate of increase of research funding to Canadian universities during the past 3 years has been far greater from private industry than from government sources. Yet primary care researchers have participated only to a small degree in this increased funding.

Development of Industry Research Ideas

Although there is some variation in the organizational structure of pharmaceutical companies and the way decisions are made about clinical research directions, in general these decisions involve consideration of the possibilities suggested by previous in-house laboratory and animal model research. Research ideas germinate from within the company as natural steps in the process of developing potential new therapies. However, even at the early stages, marketing considerations must be considered. For example, it might be quite possible to develop another nonsteroidal anti-inflammatory drug, but, because of the large number of such agents already available, marketing considerations probably would advise against such a development.

Early work with potential new agents often is presented at medical meetings and in specialized journals. Such announcements can result in a company being approached by an independent researcher who expresses an interest in studying the new agent. In other instances a researcher may be approached by the company and asked to undertake a particular project; this individual will have a good track record of executing drug trials and may have done work for the company in the past. Less commonly, an independent researcher may approach the company with an idea involving a marketed drug (perhaps to examine some outcome such as quality of life or to compare it with another marketed drug).

The Process of Clinical Pharmaceutical Research

Clinical drug studies in humans are classified into four "phases" (Stolar, 1986), three carried out before a new drug can be marketed, and one afterward.

Phase I represents the first time a new drug is introduced into human beings. The purpose at this stage is to elucidate the safety of the new agent by defining its toxicological, pharmacokinetic, and pharmacological parameters. A small number of healthy adult subjects—perhaps 5 to 20—are studied, often with a few serving as controls. The study includes baseline and periodic physical and laboratory examinations. The starting dose is less than that expected to achieve any clinical activity; then, on a predetermined schedule, doses are escalated in separate groups of subjects until either the desired effect is achieved or untoward adverse effects are encountered. In some Phase I studies, such as those involving chemotherapeutic agents for cancer, because of potential toxicity and carcinogenicity, the drug is not tested in normal healthy subjects but only in patients who have failed to respond to all known effective agents.

In Phase II the goals of Phase I are continued and expanded to include the activity of the drug in actual clinical situations. These studies are conducted by experts in the management of the condition in question, who can be expected to evaluate proficiently the response of the disease process to the drug. Subjects chosen for Phase II studies have the disease in question but must be healthy in every other respect. A control group is used, and the focus of the periodic physical and laboratory examinations is determined partly by the findings of the Phase I studies. During this phase the appropriate dose and frequency of administration are determined. After its completion, the sponsoring company decides whether the results are encouraging enough to warrant the expenditure of going on.

Phase III studies must provide further evidence of safety and substantial proof of efficacy. A drug is considered to be efficacious if it has been shown to have a significant impact under ideal circumstances. The sponsoring company must prepare an *investigator's brochure,* which describes all preclinical, Phase I, and Phase II studies, including information on patient characteristics, dosages, side effects, precautions, contraindications, and so forth. Detailed protocols for individual studies then are developed on the basis of this information. The scope of Phase III studies requires that many subjects be studied, a requirement often leading to the need for multicenter trials. As clinical exposure increases, the likelihood also increases of previously undocumented side effects or idiosyncratic or allergic reactions. The successful completion of Phase III studies can satisfy the government regulatory requirements leading to the availability of the drug for marketing.

By their nature, Phase III studies that may show a drug to be efficacious in a selected population in a highly monitored situation leave many important questions unanswered. Because they are conducted on a selected monitored population for a limited period of time, important, but rare, side effects are unlikely to be identified, and issues such as compliance are not studied. Special patient groups such as pregnant women, the elderly, and patients with other concomitant conditions often are excluded from clinical trials—but frequently may be prescribed the medication in primary care. Thus evidence of the drug's effectiveness in the primary care setting is important.

Postmarketing studies, often referred to as Phase IV, can focus attention on these special groups. Some Phase IV studies may be considered as epidemiological; in these studies, comprehensive, systematic surveillance programs are directed at qualitative and quantitative aspects of drug use and can establish the beneficial as well as the harmful effects of large-scale use under real-life conditions (the drug's effectiveness). More clinical studies may address areas such as quality of life, evaluation of new uses, intensive study of nonresponders, assessment of the drug's abuse potential, and discovering and/or evaluating idiosyncratic drug toxicity or doing comparative evaluations of the use of the drug in different patient types (Pharmaceutical Manufacturers Association of Canada [PMAC], 1991; Spilker, 1986; Stolar, 1986). The design of these studies varies widely, dependent on the question being addressed.

Potential Problems in the Relationship Between the Pharmaceutical Industry and Independent Researchers

It is recognized that the study of the safety and efficacy of new therapeutic agents would be virtually impossible without close cooperation between the medical profession and the pharmaceutical industry. The principles guiding the conduct of these two groups, however, are not necessarily congruent. Both strive to save lives and ease suffering, but at another level the industry is responsible to its shareholders to be economically successful, while physicians have special responsibilities to individual patients and to society as a whole. Problems with this relationship have received attention in the medical literature (Hillman et al., 1991; Ostergaard, 1992; Thompson, 1988; Woollard, 1991).

Several potential problems are inherent in the financial support by drug companies of drug research conducted by physicians (Council on Scientific Affairs and Council on Ethical and Judicial Affairs, 1990; Petsonk, 1979):

1. Industry is more likely to choose researchers who have proven to be cooperative and encouraging in the past; more critical or skeptical investigators are unlikely to be approached repeatedly.
2. If industry supports many studies of a particular drug, the number of reports on this drug in the literature may exaggerate its importance.
3. The company often assists in a major way with the study design and protocol, especially if the investigator is inexperienced. This aid

may lead to an overemphasis on efficacy and an underemphasis on adverse effects.

4. Should the investigator allow the company to analyze the data, there may be a danger of distortion of the results.

5. Participating in a drug trial may unduly influence a physician to use that drug in practice. (Bricker, 1989, p. 1691, pointed out: "If physicians are to be their patients' best advocates, they must be able to approach each therapeutic decision unfettered by conscious or unconscious obligations.")

6. Because of the preceding considerations, excellent industry-supported research may receive biased and unfair criticism.

One hears anecdotes of problems allegedly encountered by investigators in the course of undertaking industry-sponsored research: When the results are unfavorable, the company has refused permission to publish them, or has insisted that the first report be published in a nonrefereed journal that it sponsors, or has terminated the contract with the researcher, thereby withdrawing permission to use its confidential information concerning the drug.

A different kind of problem has arisen in Phase IV, or postmarketing studies. According to Miller et al. (1985):

> A few companies have developed a new type of "clinical trial" of an already marketed drug, in which physicians are offered a sum of money for each patient enrolled in the trial supposedly to record impact and adverse events. The physician is expected to complete a brief report, which is then filed with the company's medical department . . . the trials are limited to a small number of patients, usually 5 or 10. . . . These studies are not controlled, may not include sufficient numbers of patients to be interpretable, and are not evaluated by the institutional review board, since a protocol is not required to use a marketed drug. (p. 54)

Postmarketing studies often are designed by the marketing section, rather than the research section, of the company, and often are referred to in the industry as seeding studies, clearly signifying their underlying purpose, which is to increase the drug's profile and use.

Guidelines Addressing the Relationship
Between the Industry and the Researcher

The medical community and pharmaceutical industry alike have recognized the magnitude of the above problems and have published clear guidelines covering the many aspects of the relationship between them. In Canada, this recognition has resulted in two important documents: The *Code of Marketing Practices* (PMAC, 1991) establishes guidelines directed at pharmaceutical companies; *Guidelines for an Ethical Association with the Pharmaceutical Industry* (Canadian Medical Association [CMA], 1991) is directed at physicians. In the United States, the American College of Physicians has produced a position paper dealing with this issue (1991), and the Council on Scientific Affairs and the Council on Ethical and Judicial Affairs of the American Medical Association (1990) has published a discussion and guidelines on it. The U.S. Food and Drug Administration also is addressing the problem and invites physicians with concerns or questions to contact its office (Kessler, 1991).

These documents are highly recommended to all practicing physicians, whether or not they are involved with industry-sponsored research. The following are a few comments particularly relevant to research from the Canadian publications. From the CMA document:

> The practising physician's primary obligation is towards the patient. Considerations involving the pharmaceutical industry are appropriate only insofar as they do not affect the fiduciary nature of the physician/patient relationship . . . the physician should always maintain professional autonomy, independence and commitment to the scientific method. A necessary prerequisite for . . . research activities is that . . . these activities are ethically defensible, socially responsible and scientifically valid. (CMA, 1991, pp. 3-4)

From the PMAC document, related to postmarketing studies: "All postmarketing studies shall have a clearly defined objective which is amenable to scientific review and testing. The company shall ensure that postmarketing studies are designed/approved and administered . . . in a manner analogous to the control exercised over premarketing trials" (p. 8). These documents also address physician remuneration and ethical review.

As a general guideline, the "sunshine test" was proposed during the discussions that led to the American College of Physicians document (1991). The question, Would you be willing to have these arrangements generally known? is a useful measure of the acceptability of any relationship between physician and industry.

Benefits to the Primary Care Researcher From Involvement in Pharmaceutical Industry Research

Much can be gained by the involvement of the primary care physician in industry-sponsored research. For the research novice, participation in a Phase III multicenter trial may be a way of getting a taste of what is involved in conducting a randomized drug trial. Before commencing the trial, study physicians from all participating centers usually take part in a well-developed educational orientation that includes recent developments about the disease in question: the basic science, animal experiments, and results from Phases I and II research on the drug. The rationale of the study design is explained in detail, including use of the data collection instruments. A company research coordinator is assigned to each center to assist the study physicians deal with day-to-day issues in subject recruitment, screening, avoiding losses, correct use of the data collection instruments, and how to deal with adverse events. All of this information amounts to a practical course on many aspects of planning and conducting a randomized controlled trial.

Investigators may benefit in their practice by having an early access to and experience with the drug in question. The patients taking part in the trial will benefit by having free medication during their enrollment.

A researcher with greater experience and expertise and who is involved in the project as one of the investigators may be offered access to confidential unpublished work on the drug, well-designed data collection forms, provision of prepackaged drugs and controls, data entry, the availability of research and statistical consultation, and data analysis. Under some circumstances, assistance with report preparation is offered. The arrangements may include financial assistance to attend scientific meetings to present the results. The investigators can expect reasonable financial compensation for use of facilities, expenditure of resources, and the time and effort required for the study.

For those accustomed to the time deadlines and documentation required when dealing with public funding agencies, the relationship with the funding pharmaceutical company may seem fairly relaxed. The company may have its own deadlines, perhaps related to the next stage in the drug development or to marketing plans, but can be expected to be reasonable if recruitment is delayed.

Partly as a result of recent legislation requiring that the Canadian industry devote an increased amount of resources to research, investigators may expect company acceptance and cooperation with their own special research ideas. Researchers often can piggyback their own personal projects on to the main project, especially if they get involved early in the protocol development.

What Does the Primary Care Researcher Bring to the Industry?

A problem frequently encountered by the reader of drug trial reports is the difficulty in knowing whether the results are applicable to one's own practice. Frequently investigators are university-based subspecialists undertaking research in specialty clinics or on tertiary care hospital inpatients. The patients come under their care after referral and are usually a highly selected group representing severe and advanced forms of the disease in question. Although the drug may be efficacious in the clinical trials, it must be tested in primary care to be shown to be useful and generally effective.

In relation to the study population, research conducted by primary care physicians offers a clear advantage. Their patients are unselected; they include both early and advanced cases and all degrees of severity. Because many physicians now manage their practices with computerized data base systems, they can identify easily any potential subjects with specified diagnoses, age ranges, and gender, as well as describe the patient population from which the subjects were drawn.

For the subjects, the conditions in which the trial can be conducted closely match the health care to which they are accustomed. Familiar practice personnel look after them in the trial, scheduling can often be more flexible, and their questions or concerns can be handled more expeditiously. Subjects also feel more confident that all of their health concerns can be dealt with during their study visits. They also believe (justifiably, one hopes) that their physician will keep their best interests foremost and not allow their involvement in the research to be detrimental to their welfare. Subjects are also aware that their physician will be there to care for them after the trial is over and that they will not be abandoned by the investigator. All of these factors are likely to have a positive effect on recruitment rate and subject compliance.

Finally the primary care researcher is aware of the problems facing the primary care clinician and, therefore, is likely to generate research ideas and use outcomes that are practical and relevant. The answers generated from such projects will be of use to a large segment of the medical community.

The Role of the Primary Care Researcher in Industry-Sponsored Research

What should the role of the primary care researcher be in industry-sponsored research? In light of the process of development of a new pharmaceutical, involvement in Phase I or Phase II is unlikely. However, primary care physicians can play an important role in multicenter Phase III trials by agreeing to serve as investigators for one of the centers. By enrolling their patients in the study, they are helping to ensure that drugs that may be prescribed in primary care are evaluated in a primary care population.

It is scarcely necessary, however, to point out to my colleagues that resources—*their resources*—are scarce. It is their responsibility to ensure that the proposed study is important for primary care and, even more important, that it holds an interest for them personally. Further, if they do not have the expertise to assess its scientific merit, they have the responsibility to obtain the pharmaceutical company's permission to share the study protocol with someone more knowledgeable in research design. Many important questions in primary care need answers. It is imperative that we avoid those that are trivial or that, because of design flaws, cannot provide answers.

As an increasing number of primary care professionals become skilled and experienced in research, more are seeking active roles in Phase III studies. Those who have chosen an area of special clinical interest are in a position to stay abreast of new developments of particular relevance to primary care practice. The industry should be quite receptive to a direct approach from a researcher in primary care to assist in the Phase III studies of a new product.

Ironically the most fertile and exciting area for primary care researchers may be in the often troubled area of Phase IV. "Quality of life" issues rarely are addressed in premarketing studies, but it is increasingly recognized that they are an important consideration in assessing the role of drug therapy for most conditions. Primary care researchers are ideally situated to undertake such studies, and much of the methodology is developed and is well within their areas of interest.

Also in premarketing studies the restrictive inclusion criteria often exclude many patients who will take the medication in practice: Postmarketing studies are more likely to include all patients who the physician considers would benefit from the medication. Consequently one might expect different experiences with adverse and idiosyncratic reactions, interactions with concurrent medications, and the possible need for dose modification when used in special populations.

Postmarketing surveillance for safety and effectiveness is another natural area of research in primary care. The Canadian federal government has recognized its importance and has developed a proposal for a National Postmarketing Pharmaceutical Surveillance Program (Hylnka, 1991). Should this program be adopted, physicians in the College of Family Physicians network (NaReS) or in a university-based network could undertake studies and minimize the researcher-industry relationship concerns.

A final postmarketing area that is very appropriate for primary care is that of cost-effectiveness. What is the impact of the introduction of a new drug on overall costs? With the current concerns over the rising cost of health care, many governments and insurers are asking whether the cost of a new drug can be justified by savings elsewhere in the health system.

In this chapter we have looked at the relationship between primary care practitioners and the drug industry, but the issues and opportunities are similar for the technology industry. The development of rapid in-office tests (e.g., the rapid strep test for diagnosing the presence of a streptococcus) and portable sophisticated instruments (e.g., the audioscope for hearing testing) has meant the growth of a whole new industry. As for drugs, these new technologies have to be shown to be effective in the primary care setting before widespread adoption.

There are exciting opportunities for collaborative industry-funded research in primary care. These opportunities will be fully realized only if both partners show mutual respect and adhere to high scientific standards.

References

American College of Physicians. (1991). Physicians and the pharmaceutical industry. *Annals of Internal Medicine, 112,* 624-626.

Bricker, E. M. (1989). Industrial marketing and medical ethics. *New England Journal of Medicine, 320,* 1690-1692.

Canadian Medical Association, Ad Hoc Committee on Physician-Pharmaceutical Industry Guidelines [CMA]. (1991). *Executive summary: Guidelines for an ethical association with the pharmaceutical industry.* Ottawa: Author.

Council on Scientific Affairs and Council on Ethical and Judicial Affairs. (1990). Council report: Conflicts of interest in medical center/industry research relationships. *Journal of the American Medical Association, 263,* 2790-2793.

Hillman, A. L., Eisenberg, J. M., Pauly, M. V., Bloom, B. S., Glick, H., Kinosian, B., & Schwarz, J. S. (1991). Avoiding bias in the conduct and reporting of cost-effectiveness research sponsored by pharmaceutical companies. *New England Journal of Medicine, 324,* 1362-1365.

Hylnka, J. N., Bureau of Pharmaceutical Surveillance, Drug Directorate. (1991). *Developing a national postmarketing pharmaceutical surveillance program (PPSP).* Ottawa: Health and Welfare Canada.

Kessler, D. A. (1991). Drug promotion and scientific exchange: The role of the clinical investigator. *New England Journal of Medicine, 325,* 201-203.

Miller, K., Gouveia, W. A., Barza, M., Bower, K., Curtis, L., Decker, E. L., Dorkin, H., Estes, M., Mackey, W., Marchbein, D., Meissner, C., & Miller, R. (1985). Undesirable marketing practices in the pharmaceutical industry. *New England Journal of Medicine, 313,* 54.

Ostergaard, D. J. (1992). Relationships between family physicians and the pharmaceutical industry. *Journal of Family Practice, 34,* 29-31.

Petsonk, E. L. (1979). Conflicts of interest in drug research. *New England Journal of Medicine, 301,* 335.

Pharmaceutical Manufacturers Association of Canada [PMAC]. (1991). *Code of marketing practices*. Ottawa: Author.

Ryten, E. (1991). The funding of research conducted by Canadian universities. *Forum, The Association of Canadian Medical Colleges, 24*, 1-6.

Spilker, B. (1986). *Guide to the clinical interpretation of data*. New York: Raven.

Stolar, M. H. (Ed.). (1986). *Pharmacy-coordinated investigational drug services*. Bethesda, MD: American Society of Hospital Pharmacists.

Thompson, W. G. (1988). The ethics of physician-pharmaceutical company relationships. *Canadian Medical Association Journal, 139*, 835-836.

Woollard, R. F. (1991). Snake oil and Caesar salad: The ethics of physician and pharmaceutical relationships. *Canadian Medical Association Journal, 145*, 931-933.

12 University/Community Collaboration in Primary Care Research

ANN C. MACAULAY

Introduction

The success of university/community research groups and the current development of new collaborative research in North America are a clear indication of the importance of collaboration for the future of primary care research. Collaborative research is strong because it blends the expertise and experience of each for the benefit of all. University-based researchers have training and experience in epidemiology and statistics, while community-based physicians have long-term relationships with patients and families with myriads of health issues. Universities and communities thus can work together to further research in primary care and to achieve the vision "to improve the health of individuals, families and communities through the development and dissemination of new knowledge, fitting people's needs as they relate to primary care practice, organization and education" (North American Primary Care Research Group, 1991, p. 2).

My own background includes 22 years of practice in Kahnawake, Quebec (a population of 5,500 native people), and 4 years as a staff member of the Department of Family Medicine at McGill University, in Montreal. I believe, therefore, that I have knowledge of both sides of the fence. For the last 12 years my community practice has included research in breast-feeding (Macaulay, 1981; Macaulay, Hanusaik, & Beauvais, 1989) and diabetes

(Macaulay, Montour, & Adelson, 1988; Montour & Macaulay, 1985, 1988; Montour, Macaulay, & Adelson, 1988). This experience of community-based research was one of the most rewarding parts of my medical career. In that setting, research was not just "research," but quickly became an integral part of health care, both in the office and through developing education programs for the community. This research never could have been achieved without either community support or technical help and encouragement from staff at McGill University.

University Strengths and Problems

University departments of family medicine have much to offer. Faculty who do research typically have training in epidemiology and biostatistics; research experience; easy access to computers, libraries, literature searches, and reprints; and grantsmanship and a knowledge of funding agencies. They have access to a network of research colleagues within the university, as well as nationally and internationally, to university expertise in other disciplines, and to ethics approval boards. Ideally they have departmental facilities, such as a secretary who is familiar with typing grant applications, and, with luck, even a little seed money.

All is not rosy in academia, however: Both funding and "protected time" for doing research are often extremely low. Culpepper and Franks (1983) surveyed U.S. family medicine departments and found that "common major impediments to research reported by programs included lack of faculty time (78%), lack of funding (61%), lack of equipment and supplies (48%), lack of research skills (45%) and role models (43%)" (p. 63). Lack of funding was a major problem: "Identified federal support of family medicine research represented only 0.06% of the 1980 U.S. Federal Health research budget" (p. 67). Perkoff (1985) described an emphasis on clinical and administrative responsibilities earlier in the career of family medicine faculty than in other disciplines. Concerns about the demands on time and about the need for academic physicians to find a balance between teaching, research, and clinical practice also have been echoed from Great Britain by Hooper (1990).

What, then, are the characteristics of productive researchers, their training, and their work environments? Bland and Schmitz (1986) found that the best single predictor of faculty productivity was a supportive environment. Other successful identified characteristics were a mentor relationship, a minimum of 20% to 40% time that could be protected for research, and a community of local and national colleagues. What does this mean for university/ community collaboration? It means that although some researchers have money and protected time, many do not. Maybe this lack explains why I felt rebuffed by more than one academician when I was looking for some help at the beginning of my research career. It is all too easy for community physicians to underestimate the multiple demands of the academician's teaching, clinical practice, administration, and research, especially in an atmosphere of underfunding.

Community Strengths and Problems

Community-based physicians often have the privilege of observing a patient's health and disease, both physical and emotional, over long periods of time and in the context of the family and the community. Theirs is an excellent setting for describing the natural course of illness (McWhinney, 1989) and for explaining the meaning of actions and events (Helman, 1991).

University researchers should appreciate how local community-based research can enhance local health care in the following ways:

For direct patient care. For example, the results of my breast-feeding research in Kahnawake allowed me to tailor my counseling to patients more accurately. Patients related to this advice because the results were from their own community.

As an educational tool. Explaining the diabetes research results at public information sessions and on the local radio helped Kahnawake residents understand the high prevalence of diabetes and its complications of hypertension and obesity, and most important, the link between life-style and disease. Returning research results increases community empowerment and is an educational tool that deserves more attention.

For the development of community programs. As a result of the diabetic research, Kahnawake requested increased health education to *prevent* diabetes. Today the health services, together with the schools and with expertise from McGill University, have developed an intervention program to increase the health knowledge of schoolchildren and their families. The community sees the evaluation of this program not only as "research" but also as an important natural component of a new program.

To evaluate service needs. For example, Hogg and Lafleur (1984) and Hogg and Lemelin (1986) used research to evaluate the health needs of their community to demonstrate the safety of small hospital obstetrics and the use of their emergency room.

The above examples show the very important value of research that is conducted within a community. There is an interrelationship of the university faculty, the community physician, and the community to effect research. The ideas flow in both directions among the players, so research becomes an integral part of both health knowledge and health care.

The community physician/researcher faces the classic problems of time, money, and practice organization. This professional's life typically is structured to service patients and to pay the practice overheads. Finding time for research is difficult and may require restructuring of the practice. Finances are also difficult (Hogg [1991b] acquired financial support from local community organizations and negotiated a new approach from the National Health and Research Development Program). Another stumbling block is that many community physicians feel inadequate in the research arena. My strong conviction is that these professionals have enormous expertise and intuitive feelings about their practice and the questions that arise from patient care. They should consider the university researcher as they do any other consultant.

No one feels ashamed to call a specialist for definitive action or diagnostic help for a clinical problem; using research consultants is just the same. And remember that research problems frequently will be undifferentiated. Do not apologize for unrefined ideas! As with other consultants, it takes time to build up a good working relationship, and indeed some relationships are never satisfactory. In the case of our study of diabetic complications in Kahnawake, we planned to use a chart review, and for this we had defined *coronary artery disease* as a charted diagnosis of coronary artery by-pass surgery, myocardial infarction, or angina. Our first consultant was emphatic that we could "not trust our charts" and recommended standardized ECGs on both subjects and control groups. We changed consultants because we did not wish to undertake an invasive study. We planned a lifetime of research with this community and wished to maintain good relationships with it.

Rules for Collaboration

GUIDELINES FOR THE UNIVERSITY RESEARCHER

1. If the idea comes from the community physician, do not alter it and do not try to impose your interests. Confine your efforts to helping answer the practitioner's question. If the community physician is a neophyte researcher, make sure you spend time to explain the needs for strict methodology.
2. From the beginning, be sure there is a clear understanding of authorship rights, editorial rights, identity of the principal investigator, and your tasks as a consultant.
3. Try to gain a true understanding of the strengths of the community physician and start this understanding by traveling to meet in his or her office and visiting the practice.
4. Only assist in projects that seek funding, no matter how little this funding, but be prepared to work for free until funding is achieved.
5. Do not get involved unless you think the project is well founded, you think it worthwhile, and you think the community-based physician is committed enough to finish it. Be prepared to walk away from any project that is not catching on and that does not have the support of the practitioner's other partners or of the community itself.
6. If the research idea is yours and you are asking community-based physicians to help collect your data, you must involve them early enough so that they feel some ownership. Listen to their opinions and be easily available for ongoing communication. It is very important that the project be as unintrusive as possible in their practice setting (Borgiel et al., 1989; Hickner, 1991).

GUIDELINES FOR THE COMMUNITY PHYSICIAN

1. Start now. All you need is a question and a practice, but do research that is best done in a community setting. Some of the best research questions are small and simple; indeed, that is the best

way to start. Consider starting with observation and description of a clinical problem or patterns of illness.

2. Discuss your project with your partners and do not pursue a project that is not well supported by them and by representatives from your community.

3. Include a liaison with a professional researcher and involve that researcher from the beginning. It is important to plan the objective and methodology at the start, as it is not possible for an investigator to sort out haphazardly collected data at the end.

4. Negotiate the nature of your collaboration in advance.

    a. If the study idea is yours, do not change it unless you want to. The university researcher can help you focus the idea, make recommendations about methodology and analysis of the results, advise on the likelihood of obtaining funding, and help prepare the request for funds.

    b. Discuss issues of authorship at the very beginning. Who will be the first author?

5. Try to get funding for your expenses for every project, no matter how small. Discuss funding issues very carefully with your collaborator and consider local sources of funding.

6. Be rigorous in your methodology: Always plan on publication. Being in the community is no excuse for poor methods. Consider the need for ethical review by using a hospital board, a nearby university, or the Canadian College of Family Physicians.

7. If data collection is tied to patient visits, this should be minimally intrusive in a busy practice. Any data recording that takes more than 20 to 30 seconds should be designed to occur outside of patient care time. If possible, tie your data collection to billing and delegate as much data collection and responsibility to your staff as possible.

8. Be careful with your time. It is better to finish one project before starting another. Finishing includes final acceptance for publication.

9. Always return your research results to your community in a manner that is understandable to them, in addition to a copy of the finished article. It is your way of thanking them. It can be unusually rewarding and is an excellent tool for community education.

10. Find mentors (Jones, Wilmot, & Fry, 1991). Mentors may be other community physicians who are undertaking research on their own, through a research network, in universities, or through the North American Primary Care Research Group, which actively supports community-based researchers.

Good recommendations covering all of the above issues, from getting started to finding funding, can be found in Howie (1989), Herbert (1989, 1991), Hogg (1991b), and Gagnon, Susak, & Goulet (1991a, 1991b).

Classic Problems
in University/Community Collaboration

1. *Lack of knowledge.* Too often there is a gap in the bridge joining the university staff and the community physicians. This is especially true if the resource person from the university is an epidemiologist-statistician rather than a family physician. In these settings the epidemiologist has no clinical background, while the community physician does not have enough statistical knowledge. There are clear advantages when the university collaborator is a family physician researcher who has both clinical and epidemiological knowledge. Now that there are more university family physician researchers, this bridge should be easier to cross.

2. *Lack of respect.* Unfortunately, even when both collaborators are family physicians, myths and superstitions still are held on each side, and tensions remain between "the ivory tower" and "the real world." At times neither has enough respect for the other. Mutual respect is the single most important ingredient in any collaborative effort.

3. *Lack of understanding.* The practical aspects of research are very different for the two sides. For the community physician, patients remain patients; but for the academician, who collects data at arm's length, patients very quickly become subjects and control groups. If the community physician is collecting data at the time of a patient's visit, the research has little impact on the patient's life; but if the research requires interviews or physical examinations, the impact is significant. Until then the physician's relationship with the patient is only that of caregiver. Now it becomes that of researcher and caregiver. It is important that the research has only a positive impact on the original doctor-patient relationship. For example, Walter, Hofman, Vaughan, and Wynder (1988) implemented a school education intervention to modify the risk factors associated with cardiovascular disease, including the monitoring of total cholesterol levels. As an academician working at a distance, I could be very interested in measuring cholesterol levels of children, especially if I knew that this would be one of the first studies of lipid

levels in this age group and that a previous study had been shown to reduce them. But working in a small community, do I believe in the importance of lipid levels enough to impose blood testing on children and to be answerable on a daily basis to their parents and grandparents? Will there be a risk of negative impact from such testing at a community level?

4. *Differences of research goals.* For researchers in academia, research is a part of life. There is a real financial need for projects to provide ongoing funding, and high pressure to publish to gain tenure and respect from colleagues. For the community-based physician, research often develops out of an organized curiosity (Eimerl, 1980) and then becomes a habit. Of course, honor and glory also are involved, but there is no pressure to publish at a steady pace or the need of research funding to make a living. After publishing our results on diabetics from Kahnawake, we had a flood of phone calls from all sorts of academicians who saw this as an ideal community for research. The majority of proposals entailed highly invasive procedures and met only the needs of the researcher. At that point we made a firm rule: The only research that we would undertake here was that which would directly benefit the community. The academicians contacting us were surprised that we refused their offers to be co-authors on "more papers."

Recommendations for Successful University/Community Collaboration

Successful university/community collaboration requires that departments of family medicine have a strong base of clinician-researchers who have both designated time and fiscal support, as well as an interest in community-based research and a system to develop and maintain clinical scholars (Young, 1988). Universities should promote part-time academic positions for community-based physicians (Morris, in press). Faculty and residents need to hear of the excitement and fulfillment of community-based research and of the concerns, questions, and realities of the community physician. In return, community physicians would learn more of the essentials of research, gain knowledge, and increase contacts. Finally students and residents should be exposed to critical appraisal and research techniques. This exposure is now fundamental, and since 1986 the Canadian College of Family Physicians examination formally tests basic research knowledge (College of Family Physicians, 1990). Ideally residents should undertake a research project during their training because this knowledge and training will give them the confidence and experience they will need should they *choose* to do research in the future.

Goals for the Future

Many examples of excellent collaboration in primary care medicine can be used for models when planning for the future. Hickner (1991) reviewed the long-standing collaborations in the United States that include the Ambulatory Sentinel Practice Network (ASPN) and the Dartmouth COOP Project. In Canada there are the National Research System (Lewis, 1989) and new research units, such as the Thames Valley Family Practice Research Unit and the Primary Care Research Unit of Sunnybrook Health Science Centre, Ontario. All of these organizations have representatives from both universities and communities, have clear objectives, and accept research ideas from both sides.

The Agency for Health Care Policy and Research (Nutting & Hibbard, 1990) recommends that primary care research is needed for patients, for practitioners, and for the clinical process. University/community collaboration can continue to answer questions that need large populations, such as the management of spontaneous abortion (Green et al., 1988), and to answer questions arising from a practitioner's own setting. University/community collaboration can be used to rediscover the value of following the nature of illness over significant lengths of time, for which the classic examples of our generations include the work of Hames (1992) and Fry (1978). We should continue to refine qualitative research and to improve the tools for health care measurement that will measure functional status, quality of health, and severity of illness. These measures will have clinical applications, as well as be useful for research. There is a need to evaluate innovative research such as the "N of 1" trial, which could be a perfect tool for the community-based physician. It also will be necessary to encourage medical journals to increase the acceptance of articles that are based on qualitative research and use innovative methodology.

Past and current experience of successful university/community collaboration has produced excellent research results that are applicable to all primary care health workers. The bridges of collaborative research are being built with strong foundations. Today there are greater numbers of university-based researchers with improving departmental infrastructure and of family medicine residents, who represent the community physicians of the future, with research techniques and experience. As both sides develop respect for each other, the classic problems may be overcome. Together we can answer our questions to help us help our patients.

References

Bland, C. J., & Schmitz, C. (1986). Characteristics of the successful researcher and implications for faculty development. *Journal of Medical Education, 61,* 22-31.

Borgiel, A. E., Dunn, E. V., Lamont, C. T., MacDonald, P. J., Evensen, M. K., Bass, M. J., Spasoff, R. A., & Williams, J. I. (1989). Recruiting family physicians as participants in research. *Family Practice, 6*(3), 168-172.

College of Family Physicians, National Research Committee. (1990). *Research objectives for certification in family medicine.* Toronto: Canadian College of Family Physicians.

Culpepper, L., & Franks, P. (1983). Family medicine research: Status at the end of the first decade. *Journal of the American Medical Association, 249*(1), 63-68.

Eimerl, T. S. (1980). Organized curiosity. *Journal of the College of General Practitioners, 3,* 246-252.

Fry, J. (1978). The contribution of research to improving a family practice. In J. H. Medalie (Ed.), *Family medicine* (pp. 269-280). Baltimore: Williams & Wilkins.

Gagnon, F. A., Susak, L. E., & Goulet, F. E. (1991a). Getting started in family practice research: Part 1: How to begin a research project. *Canadian Family Physician, 37,* 596-601, 655.

Gagnon, F. A., Susak, L. E., & Goulet, F. E. (1991b). Getting started in family practice research: Part 2: How to begin a research project. *Canadian Family Physician, 37,* 850-854, 878.

Green, L. A., Becker, L. A., Freeman, W. L., Elliott, E., Iverson, D. C., & Reed, F. M. (1988). Spontaneous abortion in primary care: A report from ASPN. *Journal of the American Board of Family Practice, 1,* 15-23.

Hames, C. G. (1992). In the eyes of the beholder: A thirty-year odyssey of research in primary care. In M. Stewart, F. Tudiver, M. J. Bass, E. V. Dunn, & P. G. Norton (Eds.), *Tools for primary care research* (pp. 1-13). Newbury Park, CA: Sage.

Helman, C. G. (1991). Research in primary care: The qualitative approach. In P. G. Norton, M. Stewart, F. Tudiver, M. J. Bass, & E. V. Dunn (Eds.), *Primary care research: Traditional and innovative approaches* (pp. 105-124). Newbury Park, CA: Sage.

Herbert, C. P. (1989). A Canadian guide to resources for family-practice research: Have faith! *Canadian Family Physician, 35,* 831-834.

Herbert, C. P. (1991). Why family practice research? *Canadian Family Physician, 37,* 335-338.

Hickner, J. (1991). Practice-based primary care research networks. In H. Hibbard, P. A. Nutting, & M. L. Grady (Eds.), *Primary care research: Theory and methods* (pp. 13-22). Rockville, MD: Agency for Health Care Policy and Research.

Hogg, W. E. (1991a). A community-based practice as a research laboratory. Part 1: Why is it important? *Canadian Family Physician, 37,* 2122-2125.

Hogg, W. E. (1991b). A community-based practice as a research laboratory. Part 2: Combining practice and research. *Canadian Family Physician, 37,* 2357-2359.

Hogg, W. E., & Lafleur, R. (1984). Emergency department medicine in a rural cottage hospital. *Canadian Family Physician, 30,* 333-338.

Hogg, W. E., & Lemelin, J. (1986). The case for small rural hospital obstetrics. *Canadian Family Physician, 32,* 2135-2139.

Hooper, J. (1990). Academic departments of general practice at the crossroads? *British Journal of General Practice, 7,* 268-269.

Howie, J. G. R. (1989). *Research in general practice* (2nd ed.). London, UK: Chapman & Hall.

Jones, R., Wilmot, J., & Fry, J. (1991). The general practice research club. *British Journal of General Practice, 41,* 380-381.

Lewis, J. (1989). NaReS: Your national research system. *Canadian Family Physician, 35,* 837-839.

Macaulay, A. C. (1981). Infant feeding and illness on an Indian reservation. *Canadian Family Physician, 27,* 963-966.

Macaulay, A. C., Hanusaik, N., & Beauvais, J. (1989). Breast-feeding in the Mohawk community of Kahnawake: Revisited and redefined. *Canadian Journal of Public Health, 80,* 177-181.

Macaulay, A. C., Montour, L. T., & Adelson, N. (1988). Prevalence of diabetic and atherosclerotic complications among Mohawk Indians of Kahnawake, PQ. *Canadian Medical Association Journal, 139,* 221-224.

McWhinney, I. R. (1989). *A textbook of family medicine.* Oxford: Oxford University Press.

Montour, L. T., & Macaulay, A. C. (1985). High prevalence rates of diabetes mellitus and hypertension on a North American Indian reservation. *Canadian Medical Association Journal, 132,* 1110-1112.

Montour, L. T., & Macaulay, A. C. (1988). Diabetes mellitus and atherosclerosis: Returning research results to the Mohawk community. *Canadian Medical Association Journal, 139,* 201-202.

Montour, L. T., Macaulay, A. C., & Adelson, N. (1988). Diabetes mellitus in Mohawks of Kahnawake, PQ: A clinical and epidemiologic description. *Canadian Medical Association Journal, 141,* 549-552.

Morris, B. A. P. (in press). Community and university: Partners in research. *Family Practice Research Journal, 12*(2).

North American Primary Care Research Group. (1991, February). *Newsletter.*

Nutting, P. A., & Hibbard, H. (Eds.). (1990). *A research agenda for primary care: Summary report of a conference.* Rockville, MD: Agency for Health Care Policy and Research.

Perkoff, G. T. (1985). The research environment in family practice. *Journal of Family Practice, 21*(5), 389-393.

Walter, H. J., Hofman, A., Vaughan, R. D., & Wynder, E. L. (1988). Modification of risk factors for coronary heart disease. *New England Journal of Medicine, 318,* 1093-1100.

Young, P. R. (1988). Collaboration in family practice. *Journal of the American Board of Family Practice, 1*(1), 75.

13 Interdisciplinary Research in Primary Care: Challenges and Solutions

JUDITH BELLE BROWN
CAROL McWILLIAM

Primary care represents a philosophy of health care delivery in a wide variety of settings. Both the breadth of context and the broad scope of physical, psychological, and social problems presented by patients require the expertise of many professionals. As McWhinney (1989, p. 343) noted, "No one profession can meet all of patients' needs, hence the need to work together in teams." To ensure alignment of primary care research with practice, we need to develop parallel research teams.

The nature of research problems encountered in the practice setting confirms the need for interdisciplinary research (Blackwell, 1986; Conrath, Dunn, & Higgins, 1983). Many problems presented by patients in primary care (e.g., chronic fatigue syndrome, headache, sexual dysfunction) fall, theoretically, into the fringe area between the physical and social sciences. Furthermore, generalists, by virtue of their practice focus, tend to conceptualize broader research questions (Herbert, 1991). Even when primary care research problems are undertaken from the perspective of one discipline, findings from such research often suggest further interdisciplinary investigation needs. Investigation, therefore, must draw on the expertise of physicians, nurses, social workers, and psychologists alike if we are to fully comprehend it.

In addition, the scope of primary care problems is often of such magnitude that team research is needed. For example, investigating the system of discharging patients to chronic care at home naturally calls for representation from more than one discipline. Research of this nature requires the expertise of the hospital discharge planner, family physicians, nurses in the hospital and community settings, and, frequently, social workers in both of these milieus.

Although interdisciplinary research has been cited in the literature for approximately 40 years, only limited use of this approach appears in the primary care research literature (Chubin, Porter, Rossini, & Connolly, 1986). Effort to move in this direction requires attention to both challenges and solutions.

The Challenges

The primary care research process, its context, and the researchers themselves all present challenges to successful interdisciplinary research. The different perspectives of practitioners and researchers constitute the first barrier to be overcome.

I. PARTICIPANTS: PARADIGMS AND PREMISES

Researchers bring different paradigms and understandings to the topic under investigation. Both quantitative and qualitative studies require researchers to operate on the premises of different fundamental assumptions, to ask different questions, to use different methods, and to anticipate different outcomes. Successful interdisciplinary research begins with understanding all participants' frames of reference.

Beyond the individual researchers' perspectives, different health professions also view health and health care differently, with each discipline bringing its own perspective on care versus cure. Professionals also bring different values regarding patient needs, the delivery of care, and the research priorities (Barnard, 1987). This frame of reference also has important implications for shaping theoretical perspectives of the research topic (e.g., biomedical vs. biopsychosocial research) and research paradigms (e.g., quantitative vs. qualitative methods).

Different perspectives may present several barriers (Wilbanks, 1979). First, substantive communication between disciplines requires time and effort on the part of all participants. For example, terms from the qualitative literature, such as *immersion, crystallization,* and *triangulation,* may be incomprehensible to the quantitatively oriented researcher, while quantitative terms, such as *multiple linear regression* and *path analysis,* may be intimidating to the qualitative researcher. Simple differences in language—for instance, describing clients versus patients or subjects versus participants—may represent roadblocks to effective interdisciplinary communication.

Second, competition, coupled with professional territorialism, may lead to niche seeking and stereotyping. Furthermore, acculturation into one's own profession may be so ingrained or so highly valued that an individual may be limited in his or her ability to participate effectively as part of an interdisciplinary team.

The way potential research team members view themselves and other participants may seriously challenge their ability to contribute to interdisciplinary research. If team members are trapped in rigid roles and are fixated on the differential prestiges that their respective disciplines represent, they will not be able to see the relevance of their colleagues' contributions (Anbar, 1986). Such a starting position can seriously undermine any interdisciplinary research effort.

The work environment of the research team members also may present challenges to the process of conducting interdisciplinary research. Physicians, nurses, social workers, and other clinicians with busy practices and clinical priorities do not bring the same allocation of time and energy to collaborative research as do colleagues whose work priorities are more directly aligned to research endeavors. Unless all participants can recognize, accept, and proceed to collaborate within these constraints, interdisciplinary research may not come to fruition.

To venture beyond one's own discipline requires certain psychological characteristics for success (Bland & Schmitz, 1986; Petrie, 1986). Interdisciplinary researchers first must feel competent in their own fields. Second, these individuals must be confident enough in their professional identities to participate comfortably outside of the security afforded by their own discipline. Third, interdisciplinary research demands both imagination and a willingness to explore the unfamiliar and the unknown. Fourth, an ability to be flexible about work habits is also important (Bland & Schmitz, 1986). Interdisciplinary research begins with special people. These individuals serve as the essential building blocks necessary to achieve successful team research processes.

II. PROCESS OPTIONS

The process of interdisciplinary research presents a further challenge, for it is important to choose the most appropriate strategy. Four contiguous options exist: consultation, coordination, cooperation, and collaboration. Each requires different commitments of time and resources by all participants.

Perhaps the most familiar approach to interdisciplinary research is *consultation*. The consultative relationship is generally a one-to-one helping relationship between a clinician interested in doing research and a research consultant (Froberg, Holloway, & Bland, 1984). The consultation process may be particularly useful when the research topic is primarily of interest to a limited number of disciplines, yet the research design or specific aspects of the project demand the expertise of others. In addition, consultation simply may be a cost-effective solution to drawing in appropriate expertise for small-scale projects proposed by individual practitioners or researchers. For example, a family physician wishing to conduct a small qualitative study on how his or her patients experience labor may consult with an experienced obstetrical nurse and a researcher who is well versed in qualitative methodology. This approach may facilitate interview schedule development and project design, thus improving the chances of the project's success.

The process of *coordination* serves as a useful strategy when researchers seek to avoid unnecessary competition or duplication in their endeavors. Coordination may permit researchers to pursue different goals independently, while taking into account a mutual agreement not to compete or conflict with each other's efforts. This coordination may exist within, as well as across, disciplines. In addition to ensuring maximum return on team members' investment of time and energy, coordination ensures that researchers are spared the frustrations and personal and professional losses that come from unknowingly competing for research funds and opportunities. For example, submission of a research proposal for a center of health promotion may have more appeal to a funding agency if it is put forward together by family medicine, nursing, social science, and ethics faculties, rather than submitted individually by each of these faculties in a competitive fashion.

The option of coordination is not without limitations, however: Different approaches may either restrict or facilitate this approach. For example, if a hierarchical organizational structure exists, professional affiliation between the coordinator and one particular discipline may unwittingly create exclusion of other disciplines that may have been interested in cooperative or collaborative research pursuits. A more collegial organizational structure is more likely to enhance a coordinator's efforts.

The process of *cooperation* entails researchers assisting one another on the basis of the need for differing expertise. This approach works well when the research question addresses the practice concerns of one discipline, but the research process requires the expertise of other disciplines to complete data collection, analysis, and/or dissemination. It also may be essential when numerous and diverse researchers are involved in pursuing different objectives of the project or when tight time frames in a project make collaboration difficult to achieve.

The cooperative strategy brings a large group together for an exchange of ideas and information. The process involves agreeing to cooperate on a particular issue. If cooperation is the option chosen, researchers may understand and endorse more general goals but are free to pursue those goals from their own discipline and/or research paradigm. Each participant works independently but symmetrically with other members to address a specific component of the research project. The principal investigator normally assumes the role of facilitating cooperative interchanges (Germain, 1984).

The final strategy, *collaboration*, moves beyond the cooperative process. In collaborating, two or more disciplines actively and continuously communicate, plan, and take action toward mutually shared goals. Collaboration may be informal or formal. In formal collaboration, communication is structured, planned, and occurs at scheduled times; an informal approach is characterized by more spontaneous interchanges initiated by any participant as needed throughout the research project (Germain, 1984).

A critical aspect of the collaborative process is the evolution and maintenance of an interdisciplinary team, a process that demands team-building effort as part of its implementation. The size, duration, and cohesiveness of the group all require attention if effective collaboration is to occur (MacDonald, 1982). Team size has implications for productiveness of effort and coherence of research outcomes; the optimal team has been reported as consisting of five or six members (MacDonald, 1982). The duration the team has worked together reflects the continuity and stability of the group and affects its readiness for collaboration. Usually teams take 2 or 3 years to attain optimal effectiveness. Group cohesiveness may be affected by the mix of junior and senior researchers, who may not be equally comfortable and competent with the research approaches to be used. Mentorship of junior researchers, along with recognition and inclusion of their strengths, helps solidify group cohesiveness (Bland & Schmitz, 1986).

To any of these approaches to the research process, each of the participants brings unique personal experiences with multidisciplinary or interdisciplinary team functioning (Germain, 1984). Those familiar with multidisciplinary approaches have been accustomed to a hierarchical structure in a team, with leadership most often provided by a physician. This approach has meant that each professional has retained a unique role with focus on relevant discipline issues. In contrast, experience with interdisciplinary teams has familiarized professionals with an integrated, comprehensive approach fostered by role-sharing, collaborative decision making, and focus on mutually agreed goals. (Sangster and Gerace, in Chapter 9 of this volume, provide an excellent example of moving beyond the traditional nurse-physician hierarchy to collaborative practice and research.)

Several challenges surround the choice of process strategy. Although, ideally, primary care practitioners might prefer to pursue collaborative interdisciplinary research, a coordinative or cooperative approach sometimes may be the only realistic option. Such compromise may severely dampen enthusiasm for team work among those who idealize collaboration or simply prefer the socialization that collaborative working relationships afford.

On the other hand, the trade-offs of collaborative work may include loss of autonomous professional functioning and role blurring. Frustration, tension, and questions about professional identity may result (Schlesinger, 1985). Furthermore, publication of collaborative research requires matching the article content with the expectations of the target journal, which is focused primarily on the interests of one discipline. This challenge may prove to be so overwhelming that further collaborative effort becomes much less appealing.

III. THE CONTEXTUAL INFLUENCE

The organizational context inevitably creates further challenges (Bland & Schmitz, 1986; Hitchcock & Buck, 1990; Perkoff, 1985; Petrie, 1986; Young, 1988). The expectations of the participants' affiliated institutions—hospital- or community-based, academic or nonacademic (Williams, Nielsen, Shovic, Stuart, & Reuss, 1986)—will influence priorities and decisions. Practitioners often are motivated to research issues that confront them in everyday practice. This approach, however, may conflict with the academic researcher's requirements for promotion and tenure. University-based research colleagues have to develop track records of focused research programs and cannot always respond flexibly to practitioners' interests. Furthermore the policy and practice of many university research offices are to refuse to recognize equal partnership of the participants in collaborative research projects (Bland & Schmitz, 1986; Saxberg, Newell, & Mar, 1986; Williams et al., 1986; Young, 1988). As a result, publishing requirements and efforts to establish a funding track record often foster competition, not collaboration. Multiple authorship and shared ownership of projects and publications may prove difficult for some researchers.

Organizational mandates and related goals and priorities may create other context-related challenges for interdisciplinary research. Political tensions may arise when researchers attempt to collaborate in both hospital and community milieus. For example, findings originating from a study of patient use of both hospital- and community-based services might increase competition between agencies for already scarce resources (McWilliam, 1992).

Organizational expectations for research outcomes also may contribute to contextual challenges. The results disseminated must make sense and be applicable to the practice setting. Academics frequently are challenged to find methods to translate findings into a language and/or action that is relevant and useful. For example, critical feminist theory is highly relevant to the academic's understanding of family violence but has little practical application for the busy family practitioner dealing with wife assault in the office setting (Brown, Lent, & Sas, 1993).

The investigator who bridges several contexts may have internal conflicts around questions of loyalty and commitment to the project. For example, the academic involved in action research may have to tackle the patient care needs of research subjects during the project. Addressing the individual's internal conflict is the first contextual challenge of the process. Sometimes participants representing various contexts are not congealed as a team and thus are not able to function collaboratively. Also the research topic may not foster collaboration simply because the stage of research question development is not yet refined to a degree that permits integration of the perspectives of various disciplines. Thus understanding the multiple dimensions of the context of the research presents an additional challenge.

The issues presented in the preceding sections become extremely complex when one considers the whole picture. Solutions must address the context, process, and participant challenges simultaneously.

Solutions

Successful interdisciplinary research requires, as the first step, developing a mutual understanding and respect (Cassell, 1986). This development creates a sound foundation for the entire research endeavor. The establishment of trust among team members is essential (Pinto & Pinto, 1990). Trust allows self-disclosure without discomfort and requires setting aside professional egos.

Trust is cultivated both in the work setting and through informal social interactions. Sharing ideas, concepts, and interests, as well as developing acquaintanceships, all contribute to building trust among team members (Taylor, 1986). Team members should expect differences, confront conflicts openly, and work toward an appropriate resolution.

Fostering appropriate resolution of differences entails open communication. Communication includes seeking as well as providing feedback on research ideas, grant submissions, and papers in progress. Active efforts at communication diminish the hierarchical framework. Findings (Pinto & Pinto, 1990) suggest that teams that are able to achieve high cooperation through such open communication can devote their time and energy to task-related issues. Such teams progress beyond resolving interpersonal difficulties among group members to such productive activities as brainstorming, progress review, information sharing, and receiving feedback.

Our experience suggests that open communication results in both junior and senior faculty having an equal voice and vote on project matters. Senior faculty serve as mentors (Bland & Schmitz, 1986; Jones, Wilmot, & Fry, 1991; Rogers, Holloway, & Miller, 1990; Stange & Hekelman, 1990), as required, with junior faculty deferring to the wisdom and experience of their senior colleagues when appropriate. Junior faculty, on the other hand, may offer established researchers fresh perspectives on research strategies.

Even when optimal conditions exist, collaborative research will require matching the various researchers' strategies to achieve success. All team members should discuss openly who is appropriately involved in any project, to what extent, and who else might be needed. Beyond this, there must be a willingness to cultivate a basic knowledge and understanding of the other participants' perspectives. This willingness includes an openness to learning about other disciplines. Although some authors (Cassell, 1986) argue that professional jargon should be eliminated, others (Anbar, 1986; MacDonald, 1982; Petrie, 1986) suggest that the greatest success comes with respect for the others' disciplines and an interest in learning one another's languages. Our experience, from project development stage through publication, supports mutual respect and learning.

When optimal conditions do not exist, project participants must weigh the benefits and trade-offs of alternative approaches. This consideration will include assessing the nature of the task; who has the major skills, motivation, and time required; who can provide the necessary continuity; whether monetary resources are adequate (Bland & Schmitz, 1986); and which participants can interact readily together as required for completion of the project (Taylor, 1986). If the assessment indicates an inability to ensure successful collaboration, then the group most appropriately may opt to use a consultation, coordination, or cooperation strategy instead.

Development of a research team is an evolutionary process. Collaboration between two or more disciplines progresses through several stages (Germain, 1984). Initially commitment to collaboration occurs at only an abstract or theoretical level, with each discipline operating within the confines of its professional role. The perceived need to preserve professional autonomy may contribute to rigid role separation and perhaps to an unconscious effort to contain personal feelings of anxiety and competitiveness. Team members all need leadership support to avoid becoming discouraged in this early phase. Openly discussing and deciding a few "ground rules" for involvement of the various participants in any one project may help. Such open discussion among researchers with different backgrounds often can stimulate new ideas that would not otherwise have evolved (Conrath et al., 1983).

As project team members begin to appreciate each others' contributions, professional boundaries tend to become less rigid, and rules for involvement become unnecessary. A central task is to establish a balance between rigid structures, which prevent synergistic activities, and extremely loose structures, which result in meandering processes and ill-defined outcomes (Taylor, 1986). Once this balance is achieved, collaborative efforts begin to reap some return on investment. This stage takes time, however, and therefore requires patience on the part of all involved, particularly for those unfamiliar with the context.

Integrated team effort reflects the transition of research from work that is based on disciplinary specialization to work that portrays a more holistic or systemic view of the research question. Conscious efforts to match team members with research problems and with one another reflect the ability to overcome language barriers and a need for individual and disciplinary prestige. At this stage, participants often experience professional development and an expanded knowledge base. Furthermore they develop a realistic and reciprocal understanding about each other that contributes to conflict management and resolution of leadership and authority issues (Taylor, 1986). Such growth creates internal conflicts, though, and requires participants to cultivate insight, self-discipline, and the ability to compromise when such compromise does not violate basic professional tenets (Schlesinger, 1985).

Solutions must come also from the institutional setting of the interdisciplinary work. In particular, administrative support for the project and peer support for the project members are essential. Real time, seed money, and appropriate accommodation are essential components (Herbert, 1989, 1991; Young, 1988). Psychological encouragement and peer recognition are key factors in facilitating ongoing team effort (Bland & Schmitz, 1986; Petrie, 1986; Rogers et al., 1990; Stange & Hekelman, 1990). University research offices and faculty department heads need to recognize each investigator's role, not only that of the first author or the principal investigator.

In one of our more interdisciplinary collaborative efforts addressing health promotion in rural areas, a nurse, a family physician, environmental engineers, and agricultural experts have all compromised their more limited discipline-focused research topics. In the process, however, we have all come to understand more radical action research methodology and more progressive strategies for health promotion. We also have learned how to collaboratively negotiate project objectives and design to fit the criteria of funding bodies that were aligned more closely to one or another discipline.

Summary

Interdisciplinary research has the potential to achieve outcomes that exceed the sum of individual participants' contributions. More holistic understandings of primary care problems can emerge from such research. Collaboration offers participants an opportunity to acquire fresh and different perspectives and serves to enhance their professional development.

Interdisciplinary research results in mutual support, intellectual stimulation, and challenge, but it does not happen on its own. It is a craft that must be practiced, refined, and applied again and again to the problems that torment primary care practitioners, regardless of their discipline, methodology, and purpose (Chubin et al., 1986). Only through such conscientious effort can we hope to address the most critical research questions of primary care.

References

Anbar, M. (1986). The "bridge scientist" and his role. In D. E. Chubin, A. L. Porter, F. A. Rossini, & T. Connolly (Eds.), *Interdisciplinary analysis and research: Theory and practice of problem-focused research and development* (pp. 155-164). Mt. Airy, MD: Lomond.

Barnard, D. (1987). The viability of the concept of a primary health care team: A view from the medical humanities. *Social Science and Medicine, 25*(6), 741-746.

Blackwell, G. W. (1986). Multidisciplinary team research. In D. E. Chubin, A. L. Porter, F. A. Rossini, & T. Connolly (Eds.), *Interdisciplinary analysis and research: Theory and practice of problem-focused research and development* (pp. 103-114). Mt. Airy, MD: Lomond.

Bland, C. J., & Schmitz, C. (1986). Characteristics of the successful researcher and implications for faculty development. *Journal of Medical Education, 61*, 22-31.

Brown, J. B., Lent, B., & Sas, G. (1993). Identifying and treating wife abuse. *Journal of Family Practice, 36*(2), 185-191.

Cassell, E. J. (1986). How does interdisciplinary work get done? In D. E. Chubin, A. L. Porter, F. A. Rossini, & T. Connolly (Eds.), *Interdisciplinary analysis and research: Theory and practice of problem-focused research and development* (pp. 339-346). Mt. Airy, MD: Lomond.

Chubin, D. E., Porter, A. L., Rossini, F. A., & Connolly, T. (Eds.). (1986). *Interdisciplinary analysis and research: Theory and practice of problem-focused research and development*. Mt. Airy, MD: Lomond.

Conrath, D. W., Dunn, E. V., & Higgins, C. A. (1983). *Evaluating telecommunications technology in medicine*. Dedham, MA: Artech House.

Froberg, D. G., Holloway, R. L., & Bland, C. J. (1984). A continuity model for research consultation in family medicine. *Journal of Family Practice, 19*(2), 221-224.

Germain, C. B. (1984). *Social work practice in health care: An ecological perspective*. New York: Free Press.

Herbert, C. P. (1989). A Canadian guide to resources for family-practice research: Have faith! *Canadian Family Physician, 35*, 831-834.

Herbert, C. P. (1991). Why family practice research? *Canadian Family Physician, 37*, 335-338.

Hitchcock, M. A., & Buck, E. L. (1990). Research roles for family physicians. *Family Medicine, 22*(3), 191-195.

Jones, R., Wilmot, J., & Fry, J. (1991). The general practice research club. *British Journal of General Practice, 41*, 380-381.

MacDonald, W. R. (1982). *The management of interdisciplinary research teams: A literature review*. A report prepared on behalf of the Department of the Environment and the Department of Agriculture, Government of Alberta, Edmonton, Alberta, Canada.

McWhinney, I. (1989). *A textbook of family medicine.* New York: Oxford University Press.

McWilliam, C. L. (1992). From hospital to home: The elderly's discharge experience. *Family Medicine, 24*(6), 457-468.

Perkoff, G. T. (1985). The research environment in family practice. *Journal of Family Practice, 21*(5), 389-393.

Petrie, H. G. (1986). Do you see what I see? The epistemology of interdisciplinary inquiry. In D. E. Chubin, A. L. Porter, F. A. Rossini, & T. Connolly (Eds.), *Interdisciplinary analysis and research: Theory and practice of problem-focused research and development* (pp. 115-130). Mt. Airy, MD: Lomond.

Pinto, M. B., & Pinto, J. K. (1990). Project team communication and cross-functional cooperation in new program development. *Journal of Product Innovation Management, 7,* 200-212.

Rogers, J. C., Holloway, R. L., & Miller, S. M. (1990). Academic mentoring and family medicine's research productivity. *Family Medicine, 22*(3), 186-190.

Saxberg, B. O., Newell, W. T., & Mar, B. W. (1986). Interdisciplinary research: A dilemma for university central administration. In D. E. Chubin, A. L. Porter, F. A. Rossini, & T. Connolly (Eds.), *Interdisciplinary analysis and research: Theory and practice of problem-focused research and development* (pp. 193-204). Mt. Airy, MD: Lomond.

Schlesinger, E. G. (1985). *Health care social work practice.* Toronto: Times Mirror/Mosby.

Stange, K. C., & Hekelman, F. P. (1990). Mentoring needs and family medicine faculty. *Family Medicine, 22*(3), 183-185.

Taylor, J. B. (1986). Building an interdisciplinary team. In D. E. Chubin, A. L. Porter, F. A. Rossini, & T. Connolly (Eds.), *Interdisciplinary analysis and research: Theory and practice of problem-focused research and development* (pp. 141-154). Mt. Airy, MD: Lomond.

Wilbanks, T. (1979, Spring). Communications between hard and soft sciences. *Oak Ridge National Laboratory Review,* pp. 24-29.

Williams, A. S., Nielsen, G. A., Shovic, H. F., Stuart, D. G., & Reuss, J. W. (1986). Impacts of large recreational developments upon semi-primitive environments. In D. E. Chubin, A. L. Porter, F. A. Rossini, & T. Connolly (Eds.), *Interdisciplinary analysis and research: Theory and practice of problem-focused research and development* (pp. 179-192). Mt. Airy, MD: Lomond.

Young, P. R. (1988). Collaboration in family practice. *Journal of the American Board of Family Practice, 1*(1), 75.

PART IV

Different Settings

Almost all of the preceding chapters have concentrated on research in the office setting. Yet there are a multitude of other settings where primary care is delivered that present unique issues for care and for research. We have chosen to concentrate on five of these in the following chapters. The areas chosen have received little attention in the literature yet are of growing importance.

In Chapter 14, Dr. Freeman presents examples of successful primary care research with First Nations communities. He discusses the problems encountered by researchers and offers solutions to deal with difficult areas such as sovereignty. In Chapter 15, Dr. Gelberg takes us to the streets of Los Angeles and the immense difficulties in researching the homeless.

In Chapter 16, Dr. Beaulieu explores the growing world of the academic primary care setting and the model teaching practice, with its frequent turnover of learners and highly published full-time faculty. She offers suggestions for building on strengths and overcoming shortcomings.

In Chapter 17, Dr. Mehr reviews the issues surrounding research on the care of the elderly living in institutional settings. For too long, improving the primary care of these individuals has been given little attention.

In the final chapter in Part IV, Dr. Edwards moves the focus to the broader community. She presents a third paradigm beyond the individual as client (Chapters 4 and 5) and the community as client (Chapter 8) to the community as partner in research. Using the example of falls in the elderly, she illustrates how this problem can be researched and affected by this approach.

The basic research methods in these different settings are similar. The core problems are similar, for example, getting an appropriate sample, ensuring respect for individual autonomy, and obtaining quality data. What is different in each setting is the appropriate solution for a problem. We hope this sampling of different settings will encourage research into these and other distinct primary care settings.

14 Research in Rural Native Communities

WILLIAM L. FREEMAN

Introduction

In North America, "First Nations" people—also called American Indians, Canadian Indians, Alaska Natives, Inuit, Native Americans, and so on—are the people who were here first, before the expansion of and domination by settlers of European origin. The issues identified in this chapter relate to a greater or less extent to First Nations peoples in other parts of the world, including the aborigines of Australia, the Ainu of northern Japan, the Laplanders of northern Scandinavia, and tribal groups in Asia.

In this chapter I introduce the variety of research studies and current issues in conducting research in this setting. I review the following issues:

Descriptions of selected successful examples of primary care research with First Nations communities
The relevance to mainstream primary care of the results of such research
Frequent problems encountered by researchers in these communities
The relevance to mainstream primary care of these problems
A brief suggestion of "Where do we go from here?"

AUTHOR'S NOTE: The opinions expressed in this chapter are those of the author and do not necessarily reflect the views of the Indian Health Service.

Examples of Primary Care Research
With First Nations Communities

In the first volume of this series, Barbara Starfield (1991) noted
the relevance to primary care research of the tools used by the
community-oriented primary care (COPC) approach: epidemiology, social sciences, and health services research. In the introduction to that volume, it was suggested that primary care research
could combine quantitative and qualitative methods to its benefit. Much successful primary care research with First Nations
communities has involved both approaches.

EPIDEMIOLOGICAL PRIMARY CARE RESEARCH

Some practices of work and recreation among First Nations
communities are different from those of the dominant society
and, accordingly, may impose health risks that also differ. Inquisi-
tive primary care practitioners may notice such differences and
prevent individual catastrophes. For example, an alert clinician
noted three cases of mesothelioma in a small pueblo community
within 18 months; this finding prompted a check for this cancer
over the preceding few years, and two more cases were found,
giving 5 deaths where .05 was expected (Driscoll, Mulligan, Schultz,
& Candelaria, 1988). A search for asbestos found that it had been
dumped nearby as industrial waste and was being used to make
Indian jewelry and to whiten the buckskin leggings and mocca-
sins for ceremonial dancing. Four of the five mesothelioma patients had been silversmiths, and all five had participated in
ceremonial dances. The pueblo governor, council, and religious
leaders warned everyone of the danger and encouraged a return
to using clay as the more traditional method of whitening leggings. Another alert family physician documented a disturbing
rate of endocervical infection with *Chlamydia trachomatis* in prenatal patients (one-third of women under 20 years of age), which
led to a recommendation for universal prenatal screening (Cullen,
Helgerson, LaRuffa, & Natividad, 1990).

    A major epidemiological study looked at type II diabetes, or
non-insulin-dependent diabetes (NIDDM), which has become
a major health problem for many First Nations communities
throughout the world, following the changes to their traditional

life-styles under the pressures of "modernization." This phenomenon has been reported most widely by longitudinal studies of the Pima Indians of the Sonoran Desert in Arizona (Knowler, Pettitt, Savage, & Bennett, 1981). There is, however, marked variation of prevalence rates of NIDDM among different communities, as documented primarily by primary care, practice-based research. These studies include reports from a single practice in a Mohawk reserve in Canada (Montour & Macaulay, 1985), a comparison of practice-based data among primary care sites in Alaska (Schraer, Lanier, Boyko, Gohdes, & Murphy, 1988), and reports on 10 reservation communities in Washington, Oregon, and Idaho (Freeman, Hosey, Diehr, & Gohdes, 1989). Such studies, along with many others on topics ranging from infant mortality to accidents to cancer, have been used to understand the patterns of disease among Native peoples, to make choices about health care resources and primary care practice emphases, and, increasingly, to inform the communities themselves about their health problems (Montour & Macaulay, 1988).

SOCIAL SCIENCE RESEARCH

Because of the cross-cultural nature of the setting, many primary care studies with First Nations communities have used social science tools. A fascinating example is the descriptive epidemiological study of alcoholism on a rural American reservation in which inhabitants are familiar with almost everyone else (Nutting et al., 1980). The community organized an anonymous panel of knowledgeable community members to rate, separately and in isolation, each community member as having or not having problems with alcohol. The prevalence rates of alcoholism generated in this way were markedly different from those derived from police records, inpatient diagnoses, or ambulatory care diagnoses. The community has used this self-assessment to make choices about its health program.

A chilling study, not done by primary care researchers but with the same methods, examined the impact of modernization on a small Canadian reserve (Shkilnyk, 1985). The independent variables included loss of hunting and fishing (both for personal use and as guides for visitors) due to industrialization, mercury pollution, and forced transfer to modern housing with violation of spiritual norms and beliefs. The dependent variables included the quantitative health statistics of fetal defects, trauma, violence, intrafamilial abuse, and suicide, and the qualitative explanatory interviews with subjects.

HEALTH SERVICES RESEARCH

The patterns of morbidity and mortality in First Nations communities, which often differ from those in the dominant society, along with the rural nature and limited resources of these communities, have fostered research about different methods to deliver health care. The increased role of nurses has been noted in both Canada and the United States. Even more interesting has been the role in both countries of community health representatives (CHRs), community health aides (CHAs), and village health workers (in Alaska)—community people with special training to be an interface between the medical care system and the community. An intervention study in primary care addressed the high infant mortality from gastroenteritis in the hot, arid southwestern United States. Examining the problem in detail led to a set of changes that included low-technology preventions and treatments by CHRs; these changes dramatically reduced the mortality rates (Nutting, Strotz, & Shorr, 1975).

Obstetrical care is problematic for rural areas in general, and even more so for some First Nations communities that are particularly isolated. In the Queen Charlotte Islands in British Columbia, family practitioners examined their own obstetrical practice results for safety and outcome (Grzybowski, Cadesky, & Hogg, 1991). They found that providing full primary obstetrical care themselves, with recognition and immediate transfer of emergencies to obstetrician specialists on the mainland, led to results as good as any in the province, and probably better than would have been achieved by attempted transfer of all women thought to have risky pregnancies late in the third trimester.

Providing care to a community in a cross-cultural setting has prompted some researchers to assess the match between the health services provided and the culture of the community from a COPC point of view. For instance, a recent study compared the community-based Pap-screening rates of Native women with those of non-Natives in a practice in the Queen Charlotte Islands

(Calam, Bass, & Deagle, 1992) and found that the percentage of the Native women adequately screened was lower in every age group. The authors discussed the reasons for this difference and gave culture-specific recommendations to improve the rates for the Native women.

Another study took advantage of a "natural experiment," in which different health care delivery systems were serving different communities (Freeman, 1987), to compare community-based Pap-screening rates on two reservations involving the same American Indian group in northwest Washington State. One was served by an established fee-for-service practice that was a community clinical unit for a university's Department of Family Medicine, the other by the salaried staff of an Indian Health Service (IHS) clinic. In the early and mid-1970s, the fee-for-service practice had a Pap emphasis program in place, managed by an office nurse; inadvertently, due to shifting responsibilities, this program was discontinued in 1978. The IHS clinic had no such program until late 1977, when it started one. Community-based screening rates for the two sites were compared for the periods 1974 to 1976, and 1978 to 1980. The rates in both practices without the nurse-managed program were about 45%, and with it were about 70%. This natural crossover quasi experiment ruled out changes due to general background changes affecting both sites. One conclusion was that the economic basis of the primary care practices had little influence on Pap rates, while practice organization was the major determinant.

Relevance to Other Primary Care Research

At first glance, primary care research with First Nations communities in North America may seem relevant only to care and research with other First Nations peoples. My thesis is that such research is widely relevant.

Primary care research in First Nations communities has certain advantages often lacking in other sites. In the IHS, the total population base is known fairly well, which allows an accurate denominator in calculating incidence and prevalence rates. In Canada, especially in sites that are isolated and use only one medical source of care, the denominator is the total community.

A prime example of how research with First Nations communities can be similar to other studies is the research about diabetes among the Pima, which led to a major NIH study on the epidemiology and pathophysiology of Type II diabetes (Pettitt, Knowler, Lisse, & Bennett, 1980). The subsequent WHO diagnostic criteria for NIDDM were based largely on these longitudinal epidemiological studies of glucose tolerance and intolerance and on studies that looked at above what antecedent serum glucose levels diabetic retinopathy and nephropathy developed. It generally is agreed that the external validity of the results among the Pima extends to all people.

More often, however, it is more valuable to emphasize the differences. The examples of research given above suggest two important conclusions. First, individual communities of North American First Nations peoples are not alike: There is variation, often marked, among them. Second, many of these communities differ from the dominant society in their diseases and health care delivery systems. This variation permits "quasi experimental research," in which one can examine the same condition in different settings to see how variation of the independent variables (such as health care system, genetics, culture, or disease rates) affects the item of interest. This procedure enables one to assess conventional wisdoms, to see whether the wisdom applies only to dominant society communities or to differing communities as well.

For instance, is breast cancer screening by mammography always useful and cost-effective? Perhaps not in some groups in the southwestern American Indian communities, where incidence rates of breast cancer are low and survival rates within each stage of the disease at presentation are also low. A utility analysis of the data suggested that improving primary medical care to improve survival rates would have at least as beneficial an effect as improving mammography rates in primary care.

The research about the delivery of obstetrical services to the Haida Indians of the Queen Charlotte Islands, noted above, addressed the limits of rationalization of health service delivery systems based on biomedical concerns. Should the system *always* attempt to deliver all women with risky pregnancies in a secondary or tertiary level facility, even when those biomedical concerns conflict with patient-based concerns of acceptability and access? Is it *always* better to use physicians to deliver OB care or to use certified nurse midwives with expanded responsibilities in some settings? Is it better to use trained local family physicians to follow up cervical dysplasia or screen for diabetic retinopathy than to refer patients out to ob-gyn colposcopists, and ophthalmologists, respectively? The IHS examined these questions and found that local, empathetic, and more accessible—if less specialized—providers may be better.

Thus results of similar research in different settings can help determine the limits of the external validity of the conclusions— that is, to define to whom the conclusions apply. In the next two sections I discuss how not only the conclusions and findings but also the problems encountered can have relevance to primary care researchers of mainstream communities and care.

Problems Doing Research With First Nations Communities

A major distinguishing characteristic of the First Nations in North America is their tribal sovereignty. Given the importance of this to the social context of doing research with these communities, it is important to have at least a working understanding about it. The following brief explanation will attempt to do justice to the situation.

Tribal sovereignty has two aspects: the activities of the dominant society, and the activities of the tribal societies.

Dominant Society. Regarding the first aspect, acknowledgment of tribal sovereignty means for the dominant society to recognize and honor, as ongoing reality, the legal commitment made to the people who inhabited the North American continent when Europeans arrived. To some current observers, the phrase "First Nations" may appear to be merely a label that is "politically correct" or fashionable but is, in fact, inaccurate hyperbole. Not so, in the legal analysis of many scholars.

The European colonial governments considered the original inhabitants to constitute nations and made treaties with them. England and the United States simply were following international law of the 16th through 19th centuries; for their citizens to settle the land, the rights of these pre-European native nations to this land must first have been extinguished by treaty. Thus American and Canadian Indians *reserved* for themselves areas of their domains over which they would retain local sovereignty—the meaning of the American term *reservation* and of the Canadian *reserve* —and ceded the remainder to the more powerful nation in exchange for protection, peace, and services such as medical care. It was understood that they thereby became "dependent nations" that retained some elements of sovereignty such as self-rule but had given up other elements such as maintaining relations with other nations. Note that *sovereignty* is not a binary or dichotomous variable ("yes" or "no"), but rather a continuous one ("more" or "less").

The United States has, in general, although not fully consistently, continued to honor those original treaties and, more important, the concept of sovereignty and self-rule, *even though the nature of both tribal and the dominant societies have changed markedly over time* (Wilkinson, 1987).

Sovereignty is a major issue—sometimes *the* major issue—in many First Nations communities. The reason is that the extent of their sovereignty has been evolving for the past 25 years. Berger (1991, p. 160) noted: "In the 1970s the Supreme Court of the United States fleshed out the meaning of Indian sovereignty. In 1982 Canada amended its Constitution to recognize and affirm existing aboriginal and treaty rights."

Tribal Society. The other aspect of tribal sovereignty is what the First Nations communities do themselves to regain, maintain, and expand it. Communities on both sides of the Canadian-U.S. border are increasingly asserting their sovereignty and self-rule.

Anyone working with First Nations communities can see their assertion of self-rule without needing to be a constitutional legal expert. The intent of this overview is to point out three realities. First, the legal recognition of tribal sovereignty by the dominant society and the struggle by First Nations communities to achieve that recognition themselves foster more assertion of self-rule. Second, self-rule has legal underpinnings, in both the United States and Canada, that the wise researcher will not ignore. Third, it is often helpful in one's social relationship with First Nations peoples to at least know what the issues are.

Sovereignty, or self-rule, affects the primary care researcher in several ways. The following discussion briefly describes the problems and then suggests solutions and opportunities arising out of them.

COMMUNITY CONTROL
OF RESEARCH AND PUBLICATION

Problems. Some First Nations communities have asked, and others require, that a researcher obtain the permission of the local government before beginning any studies. Some communities have refused to give permission for one or more proposed research projects; others have required modifications of the protocol. Some have refused permission to publish results or have required modifications in the reports (May, 1989). Many researchers see these actions as restricting intellectual freedom, whereas the communities see them as ensuring they are not harmed by research or by publications that could increase the already present ostracism and prejudice against them. Researchers who get into a power struggle over whether their freedom should be restricted will likely lose.

Solutions and Opportunities. A more productive approach is to work within the political realities. Find out what the community's concerns are, because usually you can modify your protocol or edit your publications to take account of these concerns. If the local government objects to a study of the negative impact of dysfunctional families on their children, it may be saying that the research appears to be an extension of the ostracism and negative stereotypes held by many people in the dominant society. The proposal would be more likely to be reviewed favorably if it clearly is designed to obtain results that would help clinicians better care for high-risk children. Even better is to include positive research in the project: What factors helped some of the children from dysfunctional families do well? What organizations or practices in the community helped foster a good outcome in spite of the negative family environment? Documenting these factors would both benefit the high-risk children and emphasize the community's own strengths.

If objections to a publication arise out of concerns about the ostracism issue, removing the community identifier may solve the problem—for example, writing simply about "a reservation in the Southwest." If a publication reveals some private cultural practices of the community, omitting the description of the practice yet describing how finding out about them helped clinicians deliver more culturally relevant care may be acceptable. Sometimes phrasing may be insensitive; a researcher may think that he or she simply is describing a health problem, but to readers from the community the description is of their parents, sibs, children—themselves. For outsiders it is best to assume that everyone in the community is family and to use empathic, rather than blame-assigning, words.

Prevention may be better than editorial changes, however. Having community members as co-investigators or, even better, as the principal investigator helps avoid some of these pitfalls. And as part of the process of obtaining political consent, researchers should fully inform the community and its government about the proposed research and the possible content of resulting publications and negotiate respective roles. Necessary elements of information should include:

An explanation that the activity is research

An explanation of all of its purposes and objectives

An explanation of the procedures

The researchers' plans about reports to the community

The researchers' plans for publication and presentation to others and for tribal review or comment

A noncoercion disclaimer: that is, that the tribal government can give, or refuse to give, or withdraw, its permission for the research or its publication to continue

PRIVACY AND CONFIDENTIALITY

Problems. Small rural communities lack the protection of confidentiality found in larger urban areas. In urban settings the office staff and patients seldom know each other socially, and, if they do, the patients can go to another provider if concerned about loss of confidentiality; in rural areas there is often only one source of care, and staff and patients likely know each other and their families. In practice-based research about sensitive issues, patients may not trust the researcher's promise to maintain confidentiality. Worse, researchers may find that a promise of confidentiality is not kept. In rural First Nations communities, a usual practice of survey research is to have local people do surveys, but this has a disadvantage of the potential loss of trust due to the social relationships between interviewer and interviewee.

Solutions and Opportunities. The obvious response is to emphasize with the practice and research staff the importance of confidentiality, but that response may not be sufficient. Consider taking special preventive action. Role-playing with staff the conflict between the *familial* and *social* responsibilities they have as members of the community and the *professional* responsibilities they have as members of the health care team may decrease the risk of leak of information. Discussing the problem openly in a community newspaper may increase the trust of patients.

Most important, recognize that confidentiality may not be a sufficient protection. Researchers often keep identifiers as a habit, without thought. Unless it is absolutely necessary to return to the subjects or their charts later in the research protocol, make the research anonymous. Anonymity means more than omission of name, chart number, and ID such as social security number. In small rural communities, groups of demographic items, such as gender plus date of birth, or even age in years (instead of in 5-year age groups), may uniquely identify many people. In my opinion, research always should be anonymous unless you have strong justification to rely on confidentiality only.

RECRUITMENT OF RESEARCH SUBJECTS

Problems. Many researchers in First Nations communities find it difficult to recruit adequate numbers of subjects. Causes include distrust by community members of research in general, distrust or lack of understanding of the particular research project, distrust of outsiders, lack of time, and conflicting other priorities.

Solutions and Opportunities. The first "solution" is simply to accept that problems may not be entirely solvable; for instance, community members often do have more important priorities. However, you can take some steps to minimize the problem. Meeting with focus groups of community members may help modify an original research idea to be more valuable or may change the execution of the research to make it more acceptable. Meeting with the community's government and leaders in health may accomplish the same; in addition, you can ask them to help publicize and legitimize the research. The more the project belongs not just to you but also to the community, the higher the rate of recruitment. Research owned by the community is more likely to be listened to and used by its members.

CO-INVESTIGATORS AND STAFF
WHO ARE FROM THE COMMUNITY

Problems. Many community governments and residents want research projects to include their own people. The PI may be used to working with only highly trained co-investigators and staff, such as interviewers. For many of the community people involved, this will be their first research project; thus they may not have the degree of prior skill and experience the PI expects. In addition, sometimes such staff will place family, other emergencies, and community events at higher priority than accomplishing the research schedule on time.

Solutions and Opportunities. Understand that part of your role is to help train community people and to involve them in understanding the value and purpose of this research and of research in general. Although the extra time needed may be annoying, the extra effort is well worth it in terms of community support. The extra time and effort is the cost of doing business in this setting.

TIME NEEDED TO DO THE RESEARCH

Problem. Researchers used to the pace of doing their projects in other settings often underestimate by a factor of two or more the time needed to start and finish research with First Nations communities. The time needed for approval by the community and the IHS Institutional Review Board (if the IHS is involved) and to recruit staff, subjects, and others is much longer than elsewhere, in part, because neither the communities nor the IHS are research organizations.

Solution. Plan a minimum of 6 extra months.

SUBPOENA OF DATA

Problem. Subpoena of data is the nightmare fear of researchers. The raw data with identifiers of the survey of Alaska Native villagers on Prince William Sound, assessing the social impact of the *Exxon Valdez* oil spill, were subpoenaed successfully by both the State of Alaska and the Exxon Corporation. The confidentiality promised to respondents by the interviewers was violated, and future research may meet with a hostile reception. Many First Nations communities are located near sites that have potential problems with legal implications.

Solution. Research protocols that collect only anonymous, not just confidential, data protect the privacy of human subjects even if subpoenaed. This is another reason to recommend anonymity whenever possible. In the United States, non-anonymous research can be protected by Certificate of Confidentiality, given by the Department of Health and Human Services.

DISTRIBUTIVE JUSTICE

Problems. Distributive justice refers to the equitable distribution of benefits, risks, and work load in a society. Should a particular research project be done with First Nations communities at all, and, if so, should it be done in the intended community? Community governments may ask this question more frequently than in the past, due to a general distrust of the dominant society and of research in particular. Leaders may consider research that does not directly benefit their community as failing the test of distributive justice. Fortunately most primary care research does have some direct benefits to the community.

Solutions and Opportunities. Before presenting any research proposal, place yourself in the position of a community member and
ask whether it will be seen as helpful. If not, it may be better to
revise the protocol or to do the research elsewhere.

RESEARCH METHODS

Problems. Qualitative cross-cultural research has potential pitfalls. Have the instruments or techniques been validated for the
community of interest? (Validation for a different First Nations
community is generally not sufficient.) How acceptable to the
culture will the research methods and style be? Quantitative
research also has problems, perhaps more. If the study consists
of a survey, how acceptable are the questions? Problems of sample selection, transportation to the interview, prearranging for
time of interview, and time to accomplish the work may be much
more difficult than in many other settings. Even determining
who is and who is not a member of the community is not always
easy: Race may be misclassified in vital statistics, and membership may differ for an individual, depending on the purpose of
definition (to lose benefits, to gain benefits, to reflect cultural
activity, etc.). Response rates may be lower than those seen in the
same research done elsewhere.

Solutions and Opportunities. Pay full attention to the methods that
ensure quality research; for example, develop a data dictionary,
pretest your instruments, pretest the research protocol in the field,
and do more intense efforts to achieve acceptable response rates.

SOCIAL REALITIES

Problems. The biggest single social reality may be a widespread
distrust of research and of researchers. The historical experiences
for that distrust may not involve you and me, but we are its
inheritors. The distrust also reflects real losses—the First Nations'
loss of control of their own destiny, the loss of health when Europeans came, the loss of community self-esteem.
    In addition, researchers may face several concrete questions:
How and when should feedback to the community be accom-

plished? Who is the community's government, and what is its procedure to consent to and approve research? Is political consent by the government sufficient, or should informal permission by a more traditional influential structure, such as elders, be sought as well? How does one avoid getting involved in factional fights? Is the community's involvement only token, and, therefore, is its consent likely to be only token as well?

Solutions and Opportunities. "Helicopter research"—by outside researchers who dropped into a foreign country or community, did their thing, and then left—was common in the past. It is no longer accepted. Partnership and involvement are expected now.

Some of these social realities may be unavoidable. However, they usually are resolvable if you have a positive, long-term relationship with and commitment to the community. Established primary care practitioners who serve the community usually have the knowledge as well as the credibility and trust to resolve the problems. (A corollary is that if you are new to a community, you should attempt research with care or postpone doing it until established; collaborating with an existing research project by the community is almost always acceptable.)

Finally do research that helps resolve the losses mentioned above. The results of the study should help the community *return* to health, *regain* control, and *improve* its self-esteem.

Relevance of These Problems for Mainstream Research

To some mainstream researchers, the problems, solutions, and opportunities described above may appear to be exclusive to work with First Nations communities. In my opinion, not so.

More groups of people are increasingly trying to assert control or influence over the research in which they are asked to participate, as the price for that participation. Representatives of organizations of people with HIV/AIDS are on NIH committees planning the protocols. Nonprofessional support organizations for such disorders as cancer, cystic fibrosis, diabetes, and deafness have begun to influence the priorities of research in those fields.

Many mainstream primary care researchers have had little experience with the self-insertion of patient and nonprofessional groups, because primary care research tends to be a "cottage industry," compared with other research (is a "small-ticket" item and does not deal much with issues that are immediately life-and-death). This lack of experience will not continue. Due to the continuation of forces pushing such activity, ranging from more education to modeling (seeing other groups do so) to distrust of authority, I predict that patients, communities, and nonprofessional organizations will assert even more control in the future and in a wider set of situations, including mainstream primary care research.

Just as the types of problems encountered in doing primary care research with First Nations communities will become a prevalent experience for mainstream primary care researchers, so will the solutions and opportunities. Researchers will not need to reinvent the wheel in isolation; they will be able to make use of what their colleagues working with First Nations communities have learned.

Where Do We Go From Here?

In this chapter I have attempted to describe some opportunities and problems for researchers working with First Nations communities. I also attempted to convince the mainstream researcher of the value of primary care research with such communities, both to the communities themselves and to the entire enterprise of primary care research. If I have succeeded, a simple but accurate answer to the question, Where do we go from here? would be, More of the same. However, that answer is not complete.

Two implications in this chapter should be made explicit. The first is in the phrase "research with First Nations communities," implying a respectful partnership. Research "on" or "about" these communities often has been the norm in the past but will become increasingly difficult to do because the communities will not permit it. That type of research also will become less accurate and valuable, due to nonparticipation by resentful and distrustful segments of the community. Canadian and American Native peoples are increasingly concerned about their sovereignty and cultural integrity and are increasingly assertive to protect themselves and their communities and cultures. The second implication is that national boundaries are irrelevant to this research. In this chapter I have purposefully mixed Canada and the United States; however, the terms and labels, location of studies, cultures, researchers, health care systems, and legal status may differ between the two countries. Unfortunately many researchers and health care people, especially those of us south of the border, know little of work done in the other country. Primary care researchers will have to cross, indeed ignore, the border. We can double or triple the number of natural laboratories by being binational or, even better, non-national and attend to and promote primary care research with First Peoples throughout the world.

References

Berger, T. R. (1991). *A long and terrible shadow: White values, native rights in the Americas 1492-1992.* Vancouver: Douglas & McIntyre.

Calam, B., Bass, M., & Deagle, G. (1992). Pap smear screening rates. *Canadian Family Physician, 38,* 1103-1109.

Cullen, T. A., Helgerson, S. D., LaRuffa, T., & Natividad, B. (1990). *Chlamydia trachomatis* infection in Native American women in a southwestern tribe. *Journal of Family Practice, 31,* 552-553.

Driscoll, R. J., Mulligan, W. J., Schultz, D., & Candelaria, A. (1988). Malignant mesothelioma: A cluster in a Native American pueblo. *New England Journal of Medicine, 318,* 1437-1438.

Freeman, W. L. (1987). Implementing COPC: Achieving change in a small organization. In P. A. Nutting (Ed.), *Community-oriented primary care: From principle to practice* (pp. 410-416). Washington, DC: Government Printing Office.

Freeman, W. L., Hosey, G. H., Diehr, P., & Gohdes, D. (1989). Diabetes in American Indians of Washington, Oregon, and Idaho. *Diabetes Care, 12,* 282-288.

Grzybowski, S., Cadesky, A., & Hogg, W. (1991). Rural obstetrics: A five year prospective study of the outcomes of all pregnancies in a remote northern community. *Canadian Medical Association Journal, 144,* 987-994.

Knowler, W. C., Pettitt, D. J., Savage, P. J., Bennett, P. H. (1981). Diabetes incidence in Pima Indians: Contributions of obesity and parental diabetes. *American Journal of Epidemiology, 113,* 144-156.

May, P. A. (1989). That was yesterday, and (hopefully) yesterday is gone. *American Indian and Alaska Native Mental Health Research, 2,* 71-74.

Montour, L. T., & Macaulay, A. C. (1985). High prevalence rates of diabetes mellitus and hypertension on a North American Indian reservation. *Canadian Medical Association Journal, 132,* 793-797.

Montour, L. T., & Macaulay, A. C. (1988). Diabetes mellitus and atherosclerosis: Returning research results to the community. *Canadian Medical Association Journal, 139,* 201-202.

Nutting, P. A., Carney, J. P., Greenwalt, N., Miller, L. A., LaBoueff, S., Solomon, N., Tyndall, P., Robertson, B., Tonning, B., & Rixner, J. (1980). *The health care system of the Winnebago Tribe: Application of a method to assess system performance for alcoholism.* Tucson: OHPRD/IHS.

Nutting, P. A., Strotz, C., & Shorr, G. I. (1975). Reduction of gastroenteritis morbidity in high-risk infants. *Pediatrics, 55,* 354-358.

Pettitt, D. J., Knowler, W. C., Lisse, J. R., & Bennett, P. H. (1980). Development of retinopathy and proteinuria in relation to plasma-glucose concentrations in Pima Indians. *Lancet, 2,* 1050-1052.

Schraer, C. D., Lanier, A. P., Boyko, E. J., Gohdes, D., & Murphy, N. J. (1988). Prevalence of diabetes mellitus in Alaska Eskimos, Indians, and Aleuts. *Diabetes Care, 11,* 693-700.

Shkilnyk, A. M. (1985). *A poison stronger than love: The destruction of an Ojibwa community.* New Haven, CT: Yale University Press.

Starfield, B. (1991). Innovative ways to study primary care using traditional methods. In P. G. Norton, M. Stewart, F. Tudiver, M. J. Bass, & E. V. Dunn (Eds.), *Primary care research: Traditional and innovative approaches* (pp. 26-39). Newbury Park, CA: Sage.

Wilkinson, C. F. (1987). *American Indians, time, and the law.* New Haven, CT: Yale University Press.

15 Conducting Research on the Health of Homeless Persons

LILLIAN GELBERG

Primary care practitioners, having been trained to comprehensively address the health of individuals, families, and communities, have an excellent perspective from which to study the multifaceted health problems of homeless persons. In this chapter I review some of the special aspects involved in conducting research in this area.

Health Problems and Barriers to Medical Care

Homelessness is a significant public problem that is growing in intensity and is not going to go away. Estimates of the number of homeless persons in the United States range from 250,000 (U.S. Department of Housing and Urban Development, 1989) to 3 million (Hombs & Snyder, 1982). Although the homeless are predominantly single men (51%), they also include single women (12%), unaccompanied youths (3%), and families with children (34%) (U.S. Conference of Mayors, 1991).

Although homelessness has many causes, some factors may directly result in it, such as unemployment, shortage of adequate low-income housing, personal or family life crises, increases in rent out of proportion to inflation, and reduction in public benefits. Other factors, including deinstitutionalization from public mental hospitals, substance abuse, physical disability, and over-crowded prisons and jails, may cause the loss of a home in a more indirect manner (Brickner, Scharer, Conanan, Elvy, & Savarese, 1985).

Research on the health of homeless persons has focused on mental illness and substance abuse, but efforts are needed to expand the available knowledge about their physical health problems. The homeless are particularly prone to physical illness: In one study, 39% of homeless men rated their health as poor, compared to only 21% of housed men in the same community (Fischer, Shapiro, Breakey, Anthony, & Kramer, 1986). Other studies have found that at least one-third of homeless adults have some form of physical illness (Bassuk & Rosenberg, 1988; Gelberg & Linn, 1989; Morse & Calsyn, 1986; Roth & Bean, 1986). Such a high rate of illness must be taking its toll and may well prevent some individuals from escaping their predicament. One-quarter of homeless adults report that their health prevented them from working or going to school (Robertson & Cousineau, 1986). Of homeless children, at least half have a physical illness (Wood, Valdez, Hayashi, & Shen, 1990), twice the rate for housed children.

The most common physical illnesses in this population are upper respiratory tract infections, trauma, female genito-urinary problems, hypertension, skin and ear disorders, gastrointestinal diseases, peripheral vascular disease, musculoskeletal problems, dental problems, and vision problems (Miller & Lin, 1988; Wood et al., 1990; Wright & Weber, 1987). Contagious diseases such as tuberculosis (Brickner et al., 1985) and HIV positivity (Torres, Mani, Altholz, & Brickner, 1990) are more common than in the general population. Immunization status is often inadequate, reflecting the lack of preventive health care in this population (Alperstein, Rappaport, & Flanigan, 1988; Miller & Lin, 1988; Wood et al., 1990).

The literature is scant on the family planning and obstetrical problems of homeless women, but from the few available studies on this topic, we know that only one-third use birth control (Gelberg, 1985); their pregnancy rate is two to four times higher than that of the general population (11%-24% vs. 5%) (Wright & Weber, 1987); and they are more likely to have inadequate prenatal care (56% vs. 15%) (Chavkin, Kristal, Seabron, & Guigli, 1987). Consequently they have a greater prevalence of low-birth-weight babies (Paterson & Roderick, 1990) (16% vs. 7% in the general population) and twice the rate of infant mortality (25 vs. 12 deaths per 1,000 live births) (Chavkin et al., 1987).

The homeless face substantial barriers to obtaining medical care. Half state that during the previous year they did not obtain the care they needed (Robertson & Cousineau, 1986), and once it is obtained, they often have difficulty complying with the prescribed evaluation or treatment (Brickner et al., 1985; Wright & Weber, 1987).

Role of the Primary Care Practitioner

Studies are needed to determine how the homeless life-style can be taken into consideration in designing effective treatment plans. Because primary care practitioners are the main providers of health care to this population, their clinical experience would provide a "real world" perspective from which to conduct research. They offer health services to homeless persons in a variety of settings, including traditional ones such as community health centers and emergency rooms, and less traditional ones such as outreach teams or mobile medical units that set up locations where the homeless naturally tend to congregate, such as shelters, soup lines, social service centers, or outdoor areas. Research on homeless patients is useful to study diagnosis, treatment, cost of health services, compliance with prescribed medical care, doctor-patient relationships, and medical care provider attributes and attitudes. By using community-based samples, we are able to study the prevalence and correlates of illness, use of health services (including preventive health services), and barriers to use of health services.

One area where primary care practitioners' interest could be particularly relevant is the study of risk factors for illness. The homeless may be exposed to excessive levels of the risk factors for illness that affect the general population, including the use of alcohol, illegal drugs, and cigarettes. They also may be exposed to more uncommon risk factors such as overcrowding, exposure to heat and cold, lack of personal security, selling blood for an income, sleeping in an upright position (resulting in venous stasis and its consequences), extensive walking in poorly fitting shoes, and inadequate nutrition (Brickner et al., 1985).

Primary care practitioners' broad training also is needed to assess the impact of mental illness on the physical health and use of health services by homeless persons. Among homeless adults, one-third have a substance abuse disorder and one-third have a chronic, serious psychiatric disorder such as schizophrenia, an affective disorder, or cognitive impairment. The 12% who have the dual diagnosis of mental illness and substance abuse are a most difficult group to treat (Koegel, Burnam, & Farr, 1988).

Besides being well qualified and well situated to conduct research on the homeless, the primary care practitioner may undertake this research because of a feeling of responsibility to the larger community in which he or she practices. Helping the less fortunate members of our society is an integral component of effective, compassionate primary care.

Conducting Research on the Homeless

GETTING STARTED

The homeless are considered to be a "difficult-to-study" population. Because of the complexities involved, the primary care researcher would benefit greatly by collaborating with an interdisciplinary team of researchers who have expertise in medical anthropology, biostatistics, economics, psychology, and/or sociology. In developing a research question, the literature review should include articles published not only in medicine but also in the social sciences and public policy. Agency monographs and university dissertations also should be reviewed.

In designing a study of homeless persons, sampling issues loom in the forefront. Initially the population must be defined. Depending on the definition chosen, the findings will vary greatly. Some studies have defined homeless persons as those who use services for the homeless; others have broadened the definition to include those who live in emergency shelters, outdoors, or in buildings not meant for shelter. A few studies have included in their definition persons who have unstable and uncertain forms of housing, such as those who live temporarily in a hotel or motel until their money runs out or who double up in the homes of family or friends.

The criteria for identification of homeless persons need to be established. The stereotypical ones may be relatively easy to find and distinguish—that is, those who have an unkempt or bizarre appearance or who go around talking to themselves, pushing a shopping cart, or carrying bags of belongings. However, many others do not look any different from the general population. As a result, to identify subjects for a study, it is best to use a set of screening questions such as Where did you spend last night? or Do you have a permanent home of your own that you can go to? (Gelberg & Linn, 1989; Robertson & Cousineau, 1986).

Because of the difficulty of creating a complete list from which to obtain random samples of this population, many studies have relied on convenience samples. These are less expensive and easier to conduct than probability samples but may not be representative of the population from which they were drawn. The key in such sampling schemes is to minimize selection bias. For example, data collectors could approach every person within a geographic area, beginning from one corner of the area and moving to the opposite corner (Gelberg & Linn, 1989).

With great cost and care, random sampling can be done. Several studies have conducted random samples of shelter residents (Breakey et al., 1989; Fischer et al., 1986). One team of investigators (Rossi, Wright, Fisher, & Willis, 1987) approached, in the middle of the night, every individual encountered in a sample of random blocks where the homeless tend to live. Another study (Koegel et al., 1988) proportionately sampled homeless persons from three nested sampling strata: individuals who used shelter beds, those who did not use shelter beds but did use soup lines, and those who used neither.

Including a comparison group in the study design enables one to determine how unique the homeless are in their constellation of health and access problems. The simplest way to obtain such data is to use published information on an appropriate population (Gelberg, Linn, & Rosenberg, 1988; Koegel et al., 1988; Wright & Weber, 1987), but the needed data may not always be available. The selection of a comparison group is controversial. Some researchers have used the general population, which often makes the homeless look their worst (Chavkin et al., 1987; Cohen & Sokolovsky, 1989; Fischer, 1988; Gelberg et al., 1988; Paterson & Roderick, 1990); others have used impoverished housed persons, such as residents of low-income housing (Bassuk & Rosenberg, 1988; Chavkin et al., 1987), or persons who visit welfare offices (Wood et al., 1990) or who are on public assistance (Weitzman, 1989). Such comparison groups enable one to determine whether the homeless are different from impoverished housed groups or are on the continuum of poverty in their profile.

Homeless people are not a homogeneous group but may vary geographically in their demographic characteristics. Their profile is usually most similar to the surrounding community of impoverished persons who have homes. Samples limited to one part of a city may not be generalizable to other parts, to nearby rural areas, or to cities in other parts of the country (Roth & Bean, 1986).

A study's sampling location will limit and potentially bias its findings in other ways as well. Many studies have limited their subjects to homeless persons seeking medical care in traditional or outreach medical settings. Such persons may be sicker than nonusers of health services, but, on the other hand, they may be the more resourceful ones who were able to access the system. Others have only sampled residents of emergency shelters or cheap hotels (Bassuk, Rubin, & Lauriat, 1984; Fischer et al., 1986), often because such sites are the most accessible and are relatively easy to obtain a sampling frame from. They are also particularly useful for studying homeless families, who tend to be found in such locations. However, they may lead to biased samples (Gelberg & Linn, 1989; Hannappel & Calsyn, 1989). For example, in many parts of the United States there are only enough shelter beds to house a fraction of single adults and runaway youths, and sheltered facilities often exclude persons who have severe mental illness or substance abuse. Other locations for sampling the homeless have included food distribution centers, social service or day centers, jails, abandoned buildings (where homeless youths often live in "squats"), parking lots, public facilities such as movie theaters and train stations, institutions, and outdoor areas.

The time period of data collection will affect the information obtained. To minimize the identification problem, some studies have surveyed homeless persons in the early morning hours or in the middle of the night, as this timing increases the likelihood that an approached respondent would be homeless (Rossi et al., 1987). Sampling at night or in the evenings may, in fact, be required for certain locations, such as shelters, which may close their doors to residents during the daytime.

The season of data collection also may affect findings. Homeless persons' health problems, barriers to care, and attitudes toward housing may vary with the seasons.

STUDY DESIGNS

The choice of a study design should reflect the purpose of the research. The main designs that have been employed are cross-sectional and longitudinal. The *cross-sectional* design is the easiest to conduct, and, as a result, most of the studies on homeless populations have been of this type. However, such studies are limited by their inability to determine whether an exposure preceded the outcome of interest. For example, a cross-sectional study may show an association between mental illness and homelessness but cannot determine whether mental illness preceded the homeless state or was caused by it (Gelberg & Linn, 1989; Koegel et al., 1988).

A *longitudinal* design can determine whether an exposure preceded an outcome. However, it is often difficult to find the same individual at a later point in time because of the mobility of the homeless and their lack of an address and telephone. Such research is very expensive, time-consuming, and administratively complicated. Further, loss to follow-up can reduce the effective sample size significantly (by one-quarter or more), even with extensive efforts by dedicated research staff to relocate respondents at subsequent times. This attrition can bias the results because it may be easiest to relocate persons who have more stable living situations. To succeed, this method requires interviewers who are aware of community resources, are diligent in their recontacting efforts, and are willing to "walk the streets" on a daily basis to prevent loss of contact with their panel of respondents between follow-up interview periods. To date, only a few longitudinal studies of the homeless have reported their findings (Piliavin, Sosin, & Westerfelt, 1989); however, several are currently under way.

Sources of data in studying the homeless may be primary or secondary. *Primary* sources include the questionnaire, which is potentially difficult to do with illiterate or severely mentally ill respondents (George, Shanks, & Westlake, 1991). An interview may be more time-consuming and labor-intensive to administer and may reduce the reporting of sensitive topics such as substance abuse and prison histories but will increase the likelihood that the desired information will at least be recorded. As a result, most studies of the health of the homeless have employed structured interviews. Open-ended questions, while requiring extra effort in coding, are very useful for discovering responses that would not have been expected on the basis of past findings in general populations.

Doubts have been raised about the reliability of homeless persons' self-reports. Some studies have shown that, in general, they are as reliable as other populations; however, persons with severe mental illness or substance abuse may not be able to respond reliably to questions that are complex or that require complex responses (Bahr & Houts, 1971). As a result, self-report data should be backed up by objective data such as agency reports, clinical examinations, or record reviews.

Clinical assessments of mental or physical health fill out the picture obtained by self-reports; however, they require extensive training and reliability testing of data collectors. Complete physical examinations and laboratory testing can be done in clinic settings, including mobile vans, but when conducted in public settings, must be limited to areas of the body that respect the respondent's privacy (Gelberg & Linn, 1989; Wood et al., 1990). Laboratory testing in the field is possible but requires creativity because blood needs to be centrifuged (electrical outlets usually are not readily available in beach areas) and refrigerated (a portable cooler will do). Further, carrying needles and syringes on the streets may pose some danger to the data collectors from persons who desire such equipment.

Qualitative or ethnographic data are particularly helpful for developing hypotheses and for enhancing self-report data with observations of homeless persons as they directly interact with the health system (Koegel & Gelberg, 1992). Surveying key informants, such as agency directors, also provides useful information (Mowbray, Johnson, Solarz, & Combs, 1986).

Secondary data on the health of the homeless are easier to collect than primary data, but they have their limitations. Clinic encounter forms and medical record reviews are limited to the study of users of health services and to the information recorded by providers. Substance abuse, mental illness, and relatively asymptomatic health problems are often not reported either by patients, who may be reluctant to mention such problems, or by health providers, who may be too busy dealing with the primary medical problem to do health screening. Further, it may be difficult to compare secondary data obtained from different clinics' records because record-keeping requirements may not be uniform from clinic to clinic.

Other useful secondary sources of data include social service and welfare office records, jail records (Fischer, 1988), birth or death certificates (Chavkin et al., 1987), medical examiners' reports (Hanzlick, 1987), and the national census. Most of these sources, however, are limited by their inaccurate recording of housing status. One often has to base the selection of homeless subjects on persons whose home address is down as "not listed" or is recorded as a local shelter or homeless drop-in center. For the first time, the most recent U.S. census (in 1990) did sample homeless persons.

In studies that look at the health of the homeless, it can be advantageous for a variety of reasons to use measures developed for other populations. Such measures already exist, have (one hopes) undergone validity and reliability testing, and their use enables one's findings to be compared against those found in another population. The difficulty with them is that they may not be appropriate for the homeless, and thus retesting them on this population may be required. It may be necessary to develop new measures that consider the unique life situation of homeless persons; however, efforts to test the validity, reliability, and feasibility of such measures are expensive and time-consuming.

CONDUCT OF STUDIES

Who will collect the data must be a consideration. In some studies, physicians or mental health professionals have collected the clinical data (Bassuk et al., 1984; Breakey et al., 1989) which is advantageous but costly. In my own research, I have successfully employed first-year medical students, pre-med students, and lay interviewers for this purpose. The advantage of using students is that they have an interest in learning the medical aspects of the data collection and are willing to work for a stipend; however, they are only available for extended periods of time during school vacations. Lay interviewers are more costly, and some may be anxious about and uninterested in having to perform clinical evaluations. Note that all persons who collect data from the homeless, even if only from self-reports, should be cautious about contracting contagious diseases, such as tuberculosis, HIV infection, and hepatitis. It may be wise to test data collectors for tuberculosis skin test positivity both before and during the study.

A description of the research issues on the health of the homeless would not be complete if it did not discuss the politics involved in gaining access to these respondents and to the data collected on them. Providers in community health centers who have worked hard to provide medical care to the homeless may resent outside researchers publishing their data. Further, such clinics are usually overcrowded, space is at a premium, staff are overworked and subject to burnout, and patients are moving through the system at a hectic pace. All of these factors may create a sense of fear among providers that research efforts on-site will interfere with and slow the flow of clinical activities. As a researcher, you should try to create a liaison with providers and invite them to become partners. Your study should be designed with their assistance to ensure minimal disruption of the clinic and to ensure their cooperation. Their clinical hands-on experience will often prove invaluable in developing a research question and in interpretation of the data. You should also make the local government aware of your research efforts so that they do not confront you, for example, as you are drawing blood in the outdoors. The police can be of assistance by revealing the hidden areas where homeless persons may live and by accompanying data collectors in dangerous or isolated areas.

The protection of human subjects takes on particular significance in the study of the homeless because they are already a powerless and vulnerable group. Extreme care must be taken to ensure confidentiality of the information they provide regarding their housing status and sensitive subjects such as substance abuse, mental illness, and criminal history. In light of their impoverished status, care must be taken to avoid monetary or other incentives that would be so great as to be considered coercive. Finally the researcher has an ethical obligation to refer respondents with abnormal findings for health care. Because laboratory results may not be known until days after a contact is made, there must be several contingency plans for relocating cases with abnormal results. As a result of all of these human subjects' issues, ethical review is often lengthy, and enough time must be allowed to complete this effort before commencement of the study. It is useful to work directly with a staff member of the ethical review board team during the development of the informed consent process.

A major ethical issue involves the limitations that many researchers and advocates experience in applying the results of studies. The NIMBY (Not In My Back Yard) syndrome and lack of social welfare and health care funds may prevent the actualization of research findings. Researchers have an ethical obligation to mobilize efforts to ensure that their findings are heard by policymakers or health planners. The homeless themselves could be empowered to obtain the health services they need. In addition, although most researchers of the homeless do this work because they are concerned and sensitive about the plight of the homeless, they still have to be willing to report findings that may make the homeless appear negative or undesirable.

To conduct research on the homeless, funds of some sort are needed. Sources include the federal government, local government, and private foundations. The difficulty with the former is an extensive application process, a review that takes months to years (with revisions and reapplication), and the time-consuming reporting of the status of the project. Because one-third of homeless men in the United States are veterans, the VA is also a good source of research funds. Big grants, though prestigious, are not necessary to conduct research and may actually slow the research effort. Smaller studies may require the same effort of the researcher but are less costly, require less administration effort (but more direct data collection work by the investigators), may be more enjoyable to do, and often produce results similar to large-scale studies.

Future research on the homeless is needed in many areas: Longitudinal studies will determine the effects of housing, substance abuse, mental illness, and other factors on the health and use of health services by this population. Qualitative studies will give in-depth understanding of the nature of problems experienced by the homeless as they interact with the health care system and also may lead to insights into prevention of the homeless state. Programs must be evaluated to determine their effectiveness and to ensure that successful efforts are replicated in other locations (such work would include quality of care studies). New interventions must be designed and evaluated to improve the health status of the homeless, to ensure their access to care, to increase the number of providers caring for them, and to improve their compliance with prescribed medical treatment. Finally it remains to be determined whether "the system" will, in fact, make use of published data by modifying existing programs or developing new ones.

References

Alperstein, G., Rappaport, C., & Flanigan, J. M. (1988). Health problems of homeless children in New York City. *American Journal of Public Health, 78,* 1232-1233.

Bahr, H., & Houts, K. (1971). Can you trust a homeless man? A comparison of official records and interview responses of Bowery men. *Public Opinion Quarterly, 35,* 374-382.

Bassuk, E. L., & Rosenberg, L. (1988). Why does family homelessness occur? A case-control study. *American Journal of Public Health, 78,* 783-788.

Bassuk, E., Rubin, L., & Lauriat, A. (1984). Is homelessness a mental health problem? *American Journal of Psychiatry, 141,* 1546-1550.

Breakey, W. R., Fischer, P. J., Kramer, M., Nestadt, G., Romanoski, A. J., & Ross, A. (1989). Health and mental health problems of homeless men and women in Baltimore. *Journal of the American Medical Association, 262,* 1352-1357.

Brickner, P. W., Scharer, L. K., Conanan, B., Elvy, A., & Savarese, M. (1985). *Health care of homeless people.* New York: Springer.

Chavkin, W., Kristal, A., Seabron, C., & Guigli, P. E. (1987). The reproductive experience of women living in hotels for the homeless in New York City. *New York State Journal of Medicine, 87,* 10-13.

Cohen, C., & Sokolovsky, J. (1989). *Old men of the Bowery.* New York: Guilford.

Fischer, P. J. (1988). Criminal activity among the homeless: A study of arrests in Baltimore. *Hospital and Community Psychiatry, 39,* 46-51.

Fischer, P. J., Shapiro, S., Breakey, W. R., Anthony, J. C., & Kramer, M. (1986). Mental health and social characteristics of the homeless: A survey of mission users. *American Journal of Public Health, 76,* 519-524.

Gelberg, L. (1985). *Health of the homeless.* Unpublished manuscript.

Gelberg, L., & Linn, L. S. (1989). Assessing the physical health of homeless adults. *Journal of the American Medical Association, 262,* 1973-1979.

Gelberg, L., Linn, L. S., & Rosenberg, D. J. (1988). Dental health of homeless adults. *Special Care in Dentistry, 8,* 167-172.

George, S. L., Shanks, N. J., & Westlake, L. (1991). Census of single homeless people in Sheffield. *British Medical Journal, 302*, 1387-1389.

Hannappel, M., & Calsyn, R. J. (1989). Mental illness in homeless men: A comparison of shelter and street samples. *Journal of Community Psychiatry, 17*, 304-310.

Hanzlick, R. (1987). Deaths among the homeless: Atlanta, Georgia. *Morbidity and Mortality Weekly Reports, 36*, 297-299.

Hombs, M. E., & Snyder, M. (1982). *Homeless in America: A forced march to nowhere.* Washington, DC: Community for Creative Nonviolence.

Koegel, P., Burnam, M. A., & Farr, R. K. (1988). The prevalence of specific psychiatric disorders among homeless individuals in the inner-city of Los Angeles. *Archives of General Psychiatry, 45*, 1085-1092.

Koegel, P., & Gelberg, L. (1992). *Patient-oriented approach to providing care to homeless persons.* New York: Springer.

Miller, D. S., & Lin, E. H. (1988). Children in sheltered homeless families: Reported health status and use of health services. *Pediatrics, 81*, 668-673.

Morse, G., & Calsyn, R. J. (1986). Mentally disturbed homeless people in St. Louis: Needy, willing, but underserved. *International Journal of Mental Health, 14*, 74-94.

Mowbray, C. T., Johnson, V. S., Solarz, A., & Combs, C. J. (1986). *Mental health and homelessness in Detroit: A research study.* Detroit: Michigan Department of Mental Health.

Paterson, C. M., & Roderick, P. (1990). Obstetric outcome in homeless women. *British Medical Journal, 301*, 263-266.

Piliavin, I., Sosin, M., & Westerfelt, H. (1989, February). *Stayers and leavers among the homeless: Some recent findings.* Paper presented at the Homelessness, Alcohol, and Other Drugs Conference, San Diego, CA.

Robertson, M. J., & Cousineau, M. R. (1986). Health status and access to health services among the urban homeless. *American Journal of Public Health, 76*, 561-563.

Rossi, P. H., Wright, J. D., Fisher, G. A., & Willis, G. (1987). The urban homeless: Estimating composition and size. *Science, 235*, 1336-1341.

Roth, D., & Bean, G. J. (1986). New perspectives on homelessness: Findings from a state-wide epidemiological study. *Hospital and Community Psychiatry, 37*, 712-719.

Torres, R. A., Mani, S., Altholz, J., & Brickner, P. W. (1990). Human immunodeficiency virus infection among homeless men in a New York City shelter. *Archives of Internal Medicine, 150*, 2030-2036.

U.S. Conference of Mayors. (1991). *A status report on hunger and homelessness in America's cities.* Washington, DC: Author.

U.S. Department of Housing and Urban Development. (1989). *The 1988 national survey of shelters for the homeless.* Washington, DC: Author.

Weitzman, B. C. (1989). Pregnancy and childbirth: Risk factors for homelessness? *Family Planning Perspectives, 21*, 175-178.

Wood, D. L., Valdez, R. B., Hayashi, T., & Shen, A. (1990). Health of homeless children and housed, poor children. *Pediatrics, 86*, 858-866.

Wright, J. D., & Weber, E. (1987). *Homelessness and health.* Washington, DC: McGraw-Hill Health Information Center.

16 Conducting Research in the Teaching Setting

MARIE-DOMINIQUE BEAULIEU

Introduction

Characteristics specific to teaching settings must be taken into account when conducting research. It may not be immediately apparent what these characteristics are—after all, unlike environments such as native communities (Chapter 14) or the streets (Chapter 15), which contain obvious differences from the traditional practice setting, the teaching setting does not present barriers to doing research. Indeed, all of the issues addressed elsewhere in this volume apply here as well. So what is it that is specific to this setting as a research milieu?

More or less implicitly, the family medicine training setting has been considered by many to be unsuited for primary care research because it does not reflect the "real" world. "I do not conduct my research in my setting," is a remark I have heard from some colleagues.

It must be acknowledged that this critical view has a basis and was essential when most teaching settings were in tertiary care hospitals. It would, of course, be unfair and simplistic to generalize it to all training milieus. Indeed, many community-based clinics are now full-fledged teaching environments as well. However, many considerations specific to *any* teaching setting have to be taken into account when planning a research project. Some pertain to the appropriateness of the milieu to answer certain types of questions, and some to the organizational aspects of implementing a study. In this chapter I discuss some of the potential impacts of various organizational and human characteristics of training clinics on those two issues and propose strategies to build on the strengths and overcome the shortcomings, bearing in mind that each setting is different.

Use of Teaching Settings in Research

To what extent and how are teaching settings used as research settings? The family medicine literature is silent on this question: No researchers have explicitly reported on their experiences. To better appreciate the situation, I reviewed all of the original research articles that appeared in 1991 in six family medicine periodicals: *Canadian Family Physician, Journal of Family Practice, Family Medicine, British Journal of General Practice, Scandinavian Journal of Primary Care,* and *British Medical Journal.* My purpose was to answer the following questions:

1. What proportion of these articles were on observations of clinical practices in teaching settings?
2. Had the authors explicitly taken into account the fact that the setting was a teaching environment?

In all, 223 articles were reviewed: 110 in the European journals and 113 in North American ones. For 85% of the articles, at least one author was affiliated with a family medicine department.

A study was considered to have been conducted in a teaching setting if at least one clinic was described as a training center staffed by residents or "trainees" in family medicine and to be clinically based if data had been gathered from patients' observations, whether from the clinic's register or files or from the patients themselves.

The proportion of clinically based articles was about 40% (92/223) in both the North American and European periodicals. However, half of these (54/92) included data obtained directly from patients. Also, only 25% (28/113) of the studies described in the three North American periodicals were conducted in whole or in part in teaching settings; in the European journals, only four articles stated clearly that they were based on observations from such a setting.

I reviewed the method, results, and discussion sections for comments on staff/resident ratio, physicians' patient load, work organization in relation to teaching and patient care, and protocol implementation by the residents. Unfortunately this survey yielded little information on my questions. The resident/staff ratio ranged between 4:1 and 6:1 in the North American teaching settings and 1:3 and 1:4 in the four British studies. Four clinical studies were based on patients who were followed solely by residents; still that was not acknowledged as a possible confounder. In only 4 of the 32 practice-based studies conducted in teaching clinics did authors discuss issues related to protocol compliance or generalizability of the results.

The first observation from this limited survey is that most of the research projects reviewed were not conducted in training settings. In the cases where this did occur, authors rarely considered the implications of the teaching setting on their findings or conclusions.

How Do the Characteristics of Teaching Settings Influence Research?

Because of the diversity of academic settings, my intention here is to offer an overview of the important issues. I consider the impact of the organizational characteristics of these settings, and that of the people working in them, on three issues: the ability to address certain research questions, implementation considerations, and ethical issues.

ORGANIZATIONAL CHARACTERISTICS

A teaching setting is usually accountable to two organizations: the university and the health care institution with which it is affiliated. The work organization within the clinic has to be considered as well.

The *university affiliation* reduces the number of stumbling blocks faced by clinician-researchers in conducting their work. It gives easier access to the three basic elements required for successful research: time, methodological expertise, and research funds. However, it can also create conflicts in the definition of a research agenda. University-affiliated clinicians may be considered to have "low-key" research questions by their research colleagues who have learned to develop their research interests according to their "fundability"—that is, the priorities of the funding sources. Conversely clinicians often consider the researchers' questions to be irrelevant to their concerns. If such questions of relevance are not addressed openly, they can become counterproductive in an effort to bring clinicians and researchers together.

The *affiliation to the health care institution* may have a great impact on the conduct of research. The clinic may be associated with a hospital, a public health center, or, more rarely, a private practice. Administrative constraints may hamper the development of structures essential to research. The job descriptions of nurses and receptionists may not specifically identify involvement in research as an authorized activity. There may be no allocated personnel to compile necessary patient and disease registers.

In addition, the diagnostic and therapeutic resources available in a clinical setting are likely to affect the patterns of practice of physicians and the results of studies on diagnostic and therapeutic strategies. Similarly studies on the process of referral and coordination of care will be affected by institutional policies.

The impact of university affiliation can only be assumed because it has not been the subject of any careful analysis. However, I can quote an interesting observation made in a survey my colleagues and I conducted among teaching and nonteaching general practitioners in the province of Quebec (Leclère, Beaulieu, & Bordage, 1989, 1990). We found that community doctors in urban areas had more difficulty in accessing resources than did physicians working in teaching settings or community doctors in rural settings.

The way the work is organized *within family medicine clinics* can decrease patient volume in the office but not necessarily the work of staff members. A common myth entertained by nonteaching physicians is that teaching settings are less busy and, hence, that there is more time for research. However, even if more time is allocated per patient during an encounter, research activities are in direct competition with teaching and patient care imperatives.

The more staff there are, the more varied their interests and the more persons there are to "convince," train, and coordinate. It may be difficult to determine who is in charge of the different aspects needed for implementation of the project.

On the plus side, the resources placed at the disposal of faculty members for supervising residents (e.g., one-way mirrors and closed-circuit cameras) can be used for research on doctor/patient relationships and on the decision-making process. These facilities are typically not available in the nonacademic setting.

HUMAN RESOURCES CHARACTERISTICS

First, let us look at *the teachers* themselves. One of the greatest resources in our teaching settings is the presence of different professionals who contribute, through their expertise, to the development of innovative approaches. Teachers also develop observational abilities, a very important asset for a researcher. But contrary to popular belief, not all professors are committed to research, and as individuals, there is every indication that they react in the same way as other doctors. As shown in several studies, they have their own beliefs, priorities, and interests. In a study conducted on the management of ankle sprains (Beaulieu, Corriveau, & Nadeau, 1986), an administrative conflict affected the enrollment of patients. In a study on the effectiveness of the introduction of health charts on improving preventive care, Battista et al. (1991) made observations that were contrary to their expectations. Out of six family medicine teaching clinics, the clinic in which there was the *least* experimental intervention demonstrated the greatest change in preventive practices. Observation of this clinic showed that one teacher was convinced of the usefulness of the health charts and that the presence of this "champion," as the authors called him, had a greater impact on the outcome of the study than any other factor. In a similar study on the effectiveness of a computerized recall system, McDonald et al. (1984) observed that teaching physicians had not responded better than the residents to a reminder intervention. In short, although teachers are more aware of research in principle, in practice it is not necessarily the case, and we can expect that they will behave just like anyone else when they are "research subjects."

The presence of *residents* is, of course, the main difference between academic and community settings. Teaching is, on the whole, favorable to the formulation of research questions. Learners are continually asking why or how things work. Residents also can be very helpful in carrying out projects: They are a ready source of personnel who can make a contribution to research planning and data collection without extra funding. In addition, exposure to the precision required to write and conduct a research protocol is often a good experience that allows them to develop a critical view of published results. A student confronted with incomprehensible scrawled notes in patient files when collecting data readily understands the importance of complete and legible medical records as a means of communication.

Residents are apprentices first and foremost, however, and research is not one of their priorities. They are not all at the same stage in their learning process, and some have problems. This variation may compromise their compliance with the research protocol. They may be less reliable observers because of their relative lack of clinical expertise. Because they do not all have the same mastery of the doctor-patient relationship, we must be careful with studies that are interested in the "healer's art." For instance, let us take the evaluation of counseling or the study of the healing process. Are patients likely to react differently simply because they know their doctor is a student? Do we ever consider eliminating or treating differently the data obtained from a resident who is having learning problems? However, the more technical are the observations or interventions required for a project, the less likely it is that those factors become an issue.

Resident turnover is a major handicap in the evaluation of continuity of care. A study based on our residents' patients showed that although it is possible to obtain a certain degree of continuity of care for a given episode, longitudinality over a 2-year period is exceptional (Beaulieu, 1991). This rarity is the real Achilles' heel of academic settings. It compromises our ability to conduct studies for which long-term observation is an essential element (natural history of illness, impact of management decisions for ill-defined conditions). It involves a multiplicity of observers for a single patient, which may compromise the quality of the data. We are in a position in which it is easier to study discontinuity than continuity of care. In fact, the multiplicity of providers in many teaching settings has made the chart an important element in the provision of continuous care. Records in teaching settings are generally quite detailed. This facilitates their use for retrospective research.

Now a word about *the patients*. Their characteristics may be related more closely to the location of the clinic than to the fact that it is a teaching clinic, at least in countries offering universal coverage for medical services. On the other hand, patients who agree to be seen in teaching clinics, and particularly those who are followed by residents, perhaps may place less importance than do other patients on the continuity of their care. They may be more nomadic and, on the whole, belong to a less privileged socioeconomic class. There are no hard data on this, but these concerns are expressed by many. Also, given the amount of time that can be devoted to one encounter and extra support persons available, I sometimes have the impression that patients with complex problems feel especially welcomed in teaching clinics. Often these are the patients many physicians term "difficult."

ETHICAL ISSUES

The "who's in charge?" phenomenon endemic to teaching settings may complicate obtaining patients' consents to participate in a research protocol. If the resident is acting as the primary care provider, but a faculty physician is the one responsible for the research, who should approach the patient? Patients approached to participate in research are entitled to know the person responsible for the research and to receive a full and accurate explanation. The protocol should state clearly who is responsible for obtaining consent, and all eligible persons should be trained. If the protocol permits a resident to obtain the patient's consent, the status of the resident should be stated clearly, and provisions should be made to assure patients that they can meet with the supervisor if they so wish.

Another ethical issue that is specific to teaching settings arises when the student or resident is the target of the research, as in an educational intervention or an observational study. It is as important to inform learners of their involvement in a research study as it is to inform patients.

Building on Strengths and Overcoming Shortcomings

Meaningful clinical studies can be conducted in family medicine teaching settings if the limitations imposed on them are taken into account in the planning and reporting. Let us not forget the strengths of these settings: access to a variety of professional and methodological expertise, infrastructures more amenable to inclusion of research activities, audiovisual resources to observe clinical work, and detailed clinical notes.

Such research has the same external validity constraints as any other research. The specific constraints may differ, but to what wider population can the results be applied is an issue in all studies. The limited survey of the literature described here revealed that potential confounders specific to teaching practices are rarely acknowledged. In addition to the patient and study characteristics that have to be described for all studies, it is also important to consider additional factors. These factors should be included both in the study execution and reporting.

Extra efforts should be planned to promote *compliance with the research protocol* by residents. This is necessary because of their relative inexperience and the fact that the project may not be perceived by them to be a priority. These efforts could include:

Running specific meetings to discuss the objectives of the study and to get feedback

Planning additional training and supervision for all of the clinical skills involved in the project

Documenting patient recruitment from the residents and giving regular feedback

Some characteristics of the *work organization in the clinic* may be important to document and report on in order to evaluate applicability to other settings. For example:

Internal rules related to responsibility and continuity of patient care (who is in charge: a team, a staff person, or a resident?)

A measure of the physicians' actual work load, rather than just a global number of providers and patients, because a large residents-to-staff ratio may wrongly give the impression that most patients are seen by trainees when the staff physicians actually absorb most of the case load

The specific diagnostic and therapeutic resources that were available

Availability of a good information system is mandatory for a teaching practice that wants to develop research. It also helps in keeping track of the patients, thereby overcoming some of the "discontinuity" of care imposed by the presence of the residents.

Finally one should not take for granted that everyone in the clinic will collaborate readily in a project just because research is part of the mandate of a university-affiliated setting. As when one seeks the collaboration of nonteaching community physicians, research questions and design should not be imposed on the persons whom you want to participate.

One of the insurances for validity is to ask the right question, considering the setting. Earlier in this chapter I gave examples of the potential impact of the characteristics of teaching settings on the appropriateness of some types of research questions. I want to conclude with a reflection of how I think family medicine teaching settings can contribute to the research agenda that Ian R. McWhinney proposed to us in the first volume of this series (McWhinney, 1991). McWhinney did not use the conventional classification to describe research fields. Instead he identified three areas in which there is much "unfinished business": the appropriate technology of primary care, "making the implicit explicit," and the "articulation of theory."

Research on the *technologies of primary care* refers to organizational technologies (e.g., preventive systems, communication systems, coordination of care) as well as to specific technologies (e.g., rapid diagnostic tests, drug therapies, nonpharmaceutical therapies). We have seen that the particularities of each of our settings may limit the generalizability of certain observations that depend much on the availability of certain resources. On the other hand, we are in a good position to evaluate specific technologies that do not depend as much on context. Finally it is only in the teaching clinic that we can evaluate the organization that combines education and patient care.

Making the implicit explicit refers to the exploration of clinical decision making in primary care and its relationship to patient outcome but could apply equally to teaching outcomes. How shall we investigate a headache or an abdominal pain, and what are effective ways of teaching this material? What is the prevalence of specific symptoms in a population? What is the natural history of many of the illnesses that we encounter in our patients? Time is required to get those answers. Although resident turnover hampers our capabilities to do long-term studies, we can ensure that structures are in place so that we can study our own patients. For example, regular chart reviews can ensure accuracy and completeness of notes. I think that we teachers do not report enough on our own and residents' work with patients. By doing so we are cutting ourselves off from our strengths: observational skills refined by our tasks as clinicians and as teachers, and the support of the audiovisual resources in our clinics. We also can contribute to research on what takes place in the office between the doctor and the patient, between the teacher and the learner, and its impact on decision making and patient outcomes. By having both residents and experienced physicians providing care, we can assess the impact of level of training on outcomes.

Finally we have *primary care's basic research,* which does not deal with animals, cells, or molecules, but with the connections between life events, human experience, and health and illness. For research that is concerned with the *meaning* of things, we need qualitative research methods, where generalizability is not so much an issue. We are in a privileged position when it comes to dealing with that sort of question. Most teaching settings involve many disciplines, each of which has a unique perspective on the patient. Family practice nurses, social workers, and public health nurses all can contribute to our understanding of the patient's experience and problems, as well as the learner's experience and problems.

The teaching setting has grown to be an important element in the training of personnel and provision of primary care. Although it presents distinct problems, it also presents untapped opportunities to study patients, disease, and the process of care. And the teaching setting presents opportunities to study students, teachers, and the learning process.

References

Battista, R. N., Williams, J. I., Boucher, J., Rosenberg, E., Stachenko, S., Adam, J., Levinton, C., & Suissa, S. (1991). Testing various methods of introducing health charts into medical records in family medicine units. *Canadian Medical Association Journal, 144,* 1469-1474.

Beaulieu, M.-D. (1991). La continuité des soins d'une cohorte de patients suivis dans un centre de soins tertiaires par des résidents de médecine familiale. *Proceedings of the 19th NAPCRG Conference, Québec, May,* 22-25.

Beaulieu, M.-D., Corriveau, C., & Nadeau, P. O. (1986). Evaluation du traitement de l'entorse externe de la cheville dans un milieu de première ligne: La radiographie est-elle essentielle? *Canadian Medical Association Journal, 32,* 552-555.

Leclère, H., Beaulieu, M.-D., & Bordage, E. (1989). Nature des difficultés de la pratique médicale: Les omnipraticiens s'expriment. *Bureau de pédagogie médicale de l'Université Laval et Département de Médecine Familiale de l'Université de Montréal, Québec.*

Leclère, H., Beaulieu, M.-D., & Bordage, G. (1990). Why are clinical problems difficult? General practitioners' opinions concerning 23 clinical problems. *Canadian Medical Association Journal, 143,* 1305-1315.

McDonald, C. J., Hui, S. L., Smith, D. M., Tierney, W., Cohen, S., Weinberger, M., & McCabe, G. (1984). Reminders to physicians from an introspective computer medical record. *Annals of Internal Medicine, 100,* 130-138.

McWhinney, I. R. (1991). Primary care research in the next twenty years. In P. G. Norton, M. Stewart, F. Tudiver, M. J. Bass, & E. V. Dunn (Eds.), *Primary care research. Traditional and innovative approaches* (pp. 1-12). Newbury Park, CA: Sage.

17 Research in Long-Term Care Settings

DAVID R. MEHR

Only 5% of those over 65 years old live in nursing homes, but the lifetime risk of an individual spending some time in nursing home care has been estimated at 43% (Kemper & Murtaugh, 1991). Residents of long-term care settings usually have a primary physician; thus, although subspecialists and social scientists have until now dominated the field, such settings provide the opportunity for a broad range of primary care research.

A major advantage of these settings is that they offer a concentration of individuals in one place. It must be recognized, however, that they pose several unique problems as well. Mental and physical dysfunction and chronic illness are pervasive in nursing homes, which make them an excellent source of subjects for investigating advanced illness, but also make them *unlikely* to be an appropriate location for studies of normal aging. Furthermore, because they contain a vulnerable population with widespread cognitive impairment, ethical issues become especially problematic.

In this chapter I discuss types of long-term care settings, issues in selecting a sample, issues in recruiting subjects, ethical issues, data sources, and a review of recent research in the field.

Types of Long-Term Care Settings

Long-term care facilities include a wide range of intensities of care. At the low end are facilities that provide some meal services and supervision of medications. In the United States this is termed *residential care, boarding home care,* or *adult foster care. Nursing home care* covers more severely disabled individuals. This care may range from "basic" care services, such as assistance with activities of daily living (ADL), to specific "skilled" services, such as wound care, rehabilitative therapy, enteral tube feeding, intravenous therapy, or even long-term ventilator therapy. Some facilities more heavily emphasize these skilled care services, whereas others may provide predominantly basic care. Some parts of North America also have institutions called chronic disease hospitals for patients requiring constant nursing care.

Boarding home or residential care facilities have been studied much less than nursing homes and thus present the opportunity for pioneering research. They may be transitional institutions from home to nursing home or may provide a long-term residence. Because residents usually must be fairly independent, they have characteristics somewhere between nursing home residents and the community-dwelling elderly, so studies that are appropriate for either of those settings might also be appropriate here.

Sampling Considerations

Selecting an appropriate sample depends on the study goal and available resources; however, beyond the usual statistical considerations, investigators must consider the types of facilities and the distinct nursing home populations. In a study of the discharge data from the 1977 National Nursing Home Survey, Keeler, Kane, and Solomon (1981) found two distinct groups: a short-stay and a long-stay population. They identified 58% of admissions as having a mean stay of 1.8 months, with substantial numbers either dying or being discharged to the community within this time. The remaining 42% were long-stay residents, who were more likely to die in the facility and had a mean stay of 2.5 years. Short-stay residents either are recovering from an acute limited condition, such as a hip fracture, or are so severely debilitated that they die soon after admission (e.g., from an advanced malignancy). A typical long-stay resident might have significant dementia or irreversible physical impairment from a stroke.

Sampling from admissions or discharges predominantly identifies short-stay residents (Wayne, Rhyne, Thompson, & Davis, 1991); however, cross-sectional samples of all residents present in a facility are weighted heavily toward long-stay residents, who constitute 91% of this population (Keeler et al., 1981). Therefore, to study, say, hip fracture rehabilitation, the researcher should seek a facility offering skilled care and use an admission sample. If the goal were to investigate nursing-home-acquired infections, either a basic care or a skilled care facility might be appropriate, and most likely one would want to sample cross-sectionally.

Characteristics of the Nursing Home Population

Nursing home residents are distinctively different from the community-dwelling elderly, and studies of long-term care residents must take into account their characteristics. The 1985 National Nursing Home Survey (Hing, 1989) includes a wealth of information about a cross-sectional sample of nursing home residents in the United States, identifying them as primarily female (72%), quite old (74% over 75), mostly widowed (61%), and significantly impaired: Only 10% were independent in the six Katz activities of daily living (ADL), and 62% were dependent in four or more ADL. Mental disorders were extremely common: 43% had a diagnosis of dementia, 62% had disorientation or memory impairment, and 38.4% had behavior problems. In addition, 42% were characterized as having a mood disturbance, and 14% were diagnosed as having a depressive disorder.

Subject Recruitment

A variety of barriers exist to the recruitment of nursing home residents as research subjects. The high frequency of residents using multiple medications and having multiple medical conditions may limit an investigator's ability to find subjects who meet specified study criteria. Staff or family may not be supportive, and the process of informed consent may be difficult.

Residents are more willing to participate in research when they believe that it is directly applicable to them (Hoffman, Marron, Fillit, & Libow, 1983; Kaye, Lawton, & Kaye, 1990). Not surprisingly, they are also less likely to consent to protocols with invasive procedures (Lipsitz, Pluchino, & Wright, 1987). Lipsitz and colleagues (1987) reported that few residents reviewed for inclusion in one of four protocols ultimately participated (between 5% for studies of vasopressin regulation and 25% for studies of bladder function and incontinence). Most exclusions were for violations of study criteria, but, except for the incontinence study, where the refusal rate was 19%, 54% to 86% of those found eligible to participate in a study declined.

Despite these difficulties, persistence on the part of the investigator can be rewarded with substantial participation rates. A randomized controlled trial of the efficacy of prompted voiding (a protocol of prompting more frequent voiding to prevent incontinence) gained informed consent to participate from 77% of 250 potential subjects and eventually was able to use 57% after exclusion of those found, after observation, not to meet the specific study criteria (Hu et al., 1989).

I have observed that nursing homes are willing to participate in research and aid in subject recruitment if appropriate relationships are established, such as building a relationship with staff and administration and providing adequate assurances concerning the protection of the privacy and rights of residents. If possible, the researchers should identify potential benefit to the residents or the facility from the investigation—for example, by providing material for mandated quality assurance activities or by defraying part of one or more employees' salaries for aiding in the study. Eish, Colling, Ouslander, Hadley, and Campbell (1991) discussed a number of ways to improve nursing home staff cooperation with implementation of even a complex study: (a) minimize disruptions of routine for both patients and nurse aides, (b) inform workers on all shifts, (c) incorporate a supportive staff member as a "consultant" to the research team, (d) use a nonthreatening approach to nurse aides, (e) provide assistance with patient personal care, (f) provide empathy concerning staff work loads, (g) provide positive reinforcement, (h) do not use the nursing home's supplies, (i) use humor in conversation, and (j) provide visual (graphic) feedback.

Ethical Issues

In long-term care research involving observations of human subjects, ethical issues require particular attention. As noted above, many nursing home residents exhibit some cognitive impairment, and most are quite dependent in ADL. Thus nursing homes contain a vulnerable population with limited capacity for decision making. Investigators and ethics review committees (institutional review boards in the United States) are particularly obligated to consider whether studies adhere to the three central ethical principles of *autonomy, beneficence,* and *distributive justice* (Cassel, 1987).

We respect an individual's *autonomy* by obtaining informed consent and ensuring the right to withdraw from a study at any time. For a potential subject to render informed consent, there must be adequate information, absence of coercion, and competence (Cassel, 1985). Where individuals are unable to understand the nature and consequences of participation in a study, a proxy, preferably indicated by advance directives or guardian status, should be contacted for consent (Annas & Glantz, 1986; Melnick, Dubler, Weisbard, & Butler, 1984; Warren et al., 1986). Even where a proxy has consented, the resident should assent to the study to the extent of not actively opposing its implementation. The ethics review committee may require a variety of procedures to ensure that consent is not coerced and that subjects with marginal competence are treated appropriately. Because of the complexities of the consent process, studies that involve recruitment of cognitively impaired individuals generally will need to allow extra time for obtaining a single consent (half an hour or more) and a longer period of time overall for subject recruitment (Eish et al., 1991).

Beneficence concerns an analysis of potential benefits and harms. Risks to subjects must be commensurate to potential benefits. Review panels often apply more rigorous standards to protocols and consent procedures in nursing homes than to research in other populations. Some have argued for very stringent standards where incompetent subjects are involved: The research problem should be unique to the population, and the study should involve either no risk or minimal risk (Annas & Glantz, 1986). Universally accepted standards have not been established; nonetheless, studies that might be acceptable in the free-living elderly may not be acceptable in the nursing home setting. Historically nursing home residents have suffered substantial abuses, including the particularly egregious example of the injection of live cancer cells into unsuspecting subjects (Beecher, 1966).

In long-term care settings, *distributive justice* concerns whether the burdens and potential rewards of research should accrue to institutional residents, as opposed to other elderly individuals. This is not an issue for studies in which the long-term care setting is a unique environment—for example, nursing-home-acquired infections or behavioral management of a group of demented residents. It is a pertinent issue, however, if the setting is simply being selected out of convenience as a way to study an elderly population. For example, research into incontinence in a nursing home setting is strongly justified if it is a different entity than is incontinence among the community-dwelling elderly.

Data Sources

Potential data sources for nursing home studies include computerized data bases, medical record review, and original data collection. Each has strengths and weaknesses. Computerized data bases exist for certain governmental studies, such as the National Nursing Home Survey (Hing, 1989). In addition, the U.S. Department of Veterans Affairs and some nursing home chains in the United States have developed large data bases of nursing home assessments. Since October 1990, completion of the congressionally mandated minimum data set (MDS) has been required for residents in nursing homes throughout the United States. The MDS contains a standard set of items concerning a variety of domains, including demographics, mental status, communication problems, sensory deficits, ADL function, continence patterns, diagnoses, conditions, treatments, and more (Morris, Hawes, Murphy, & Nonemaker, 1991). In many states this information may be computerized and available to researchers. Large data sets provide for the possibility of considering the same items over large groups of people and the evaluation of proportionately small subsets of a population. However, the investigator cannot ensure uniformity in data collection or that the items of most concern in a specific investigation are collected. In this way, large data sets may yield disappointing results.

The value of nursing home records for research, as with all medical records, depends on the quality of the reporting. This quality will vary from facility to facility, but some items may be relatively well reported in many facilities, such as information on basic functional status, medication information, periodic (usually monthly) weights and vital signs, and evidence of decubitus ulcers. In contrast, physicians' progress notes are frequently sparse, and many important therapeutic decisions are made over the telephone and never discussed in progress notes. Nursing progress notes may be somewhat more revealing but are also often quite incomplete. Vital signs may or may not be recorded at the beginning of an illness episode, and frequency of obtaining them other than for the monthly routine is often quite arbitrary. Medical record review studies that have been done have frequently focused on the use of specific medications. Medical record review has unrealized potential in the nursing home setting, particularly for exploratory studies.

Prospective data collection is potentially the best method of obtaining specific reliable information but poses several important problems. First is the question of who will collect the data. Nursing homes depend heavily on nurse aides to perform many aspects of care. Typically these workers are poorly educated, poorly paid, and have demanding responsibilities, and obtaining cooperation from them for collection of research data may be difficult or impossible. Thus a research assistant or a clinician often will be required; however, particularly in intervention studies, the introduction of outside personnel may so alter the setting as to severely limit the generalizability of study conclusions. Eish et al. (1991) attempted to address this problem in an incontinence intervention study by using nurse aides for the intervention and research assistants for data collection.

A second problem is that, in many cases, no standardized instruments exist to assess variables of interest, and even where they do, their appropriate use in the long-term care setting may be subject to controversy. No consensus exists concerning the most appropriate scale for measuring physical function or ADL in the nursing home, and all ADL scales may be relatively insensitive to change in status (Applegate, Blass, & Williams, 1990). In another example, a study of the Yesavage Geriatric Depression Scale and the Folstein Mini-Mental State Examination found the latter but not the former to be sensitive and specific in a nursing home setting (Kafonek et al., 1989).

Third, the expenses of prospective data collection in many cases will require major outside funding to pay personnel, to train them, and to supervise data collection. Very simple studies with minimal data collection may be possible, with individual clinicians collecting data on their own patients or with personnel at the nursing home participating in collecting data. Small amounts of funding may be able to defray some costs for the nursing home to encourage its participation in such an effort.

Overview of Current Nursing Home Research

I performed a MEDLINE search to identify all published research from 1987 to 1991 concerning nursing home patients in the following journals: *New England Journal of Medicine, JAMA, Archives of Internal Medicine, Annals of Internal Medicine, Journal of Family Practice, Journal of the American Board of Family Practice, Journal of the American Geriatrics Society, The Gerontologist, Journal of Gerontology, Medical Care, Health Services Research,* and *American Journal of Public Health Association.* I selected all papers with abstracts that involved patient-level data (as opposed to surveys of facilities). By using this methodology, 175 relevant studies were identified from the 5-year period. Their distribution by topic is indicated in Table 17.1.

Only a small number of these studies fall outside of the purview of primary care; however, many were performed by subspecialist researchers at academically affiliated nursing homes or at nursing homes attached to hospitals for veterans. Only eight clinical studies (labeled biomedical studies) were identified where the approach was clearly outside of the usual primary care paradigm. Nonetheless one of the major problems identified in this review of nursing home research is the question of generalizability. Just as the morbidity and the natural history of a disease may be far different in the primary care setting than in tertiary medical care centers, so investigations in community nursing homes may yield substantially different results than studies in teaching nursing homes or hospital-associated nursing homes. In short, many

Table 17.1 Nursing Home Research, 1986-1991, in 12 Selected Journals

Research Topic	Number of Papers	%
Infection	28	(16.0)
Dementia/behavior/psychosocial issues	21	(12.0)
Health services/process of care	17	(9.7)
Incontinence/catheter use and complications	15	(8.6)
Drugs	13	(7.4)
Ethics	13	(7.4)
Outcomes of care	12	(6.9)
Mobility/falls/hip fracture	11	(6.3)
Other specific illnesses and conditions	11	(6.3)
Biomedical studies	8	(4.6)
Miscellaneous	8	(4.6)
Research instruments	7	(4.0)
Nutrition	5	(2.9)
Restraint use	3	(1.7)
Research process	3	(1.7)

of the issues that are applicable to primary care research as a whole are also relevant to the long-term care setting.

Infection is an important cause of nursing home morbidity and mortality and was the leading research topic identified. Most studies concerning infection were predominantly descriptive, relating to incidence and prevalence. Several studies concerned drug-resistant microorganisms. Many of the studies were performed at institutions closely linked to tertiary acute care hospitals, which therefore may have a spectrum of infectious diseases different from those of other nursing homes.

The next largest category was dementia, behavior, and psychosocial issues. Examples of studies in this category include characterizations of individuals with dementia and depression, studies of specific behavioral interventions, and descriptions of specific social characterizations of residents. Health services research and process of care includes studies of alternative care systems, use of health services (e.g., ambulance transport to hospitals), and studies comparing different approaches to care on a facility level (e.g., the impact of nurse practitioners on care). Incontinence is a prevalent problem in nursing homes: Specific studies ranged from the appropriate approach to obtaining urine for culture from men with condom catheters, to intervention trials of prompted voiding. Drug studies focused on the use and misuse of specific medications or groups of medications in the nursing home population. Psychotropic drugs were a major area of concern, as was antibiotic use. Ethics studies predominantly examined terminal care decision making and the many ramifications of the use of advance directives. Examples include questions about how closely such directives are followed in practice, and evidence for a lack of congruence between family members and residents in the understanding of what the resident would want in hypothetical situations.

Qualitative research is rare in the nursing home literature; even a more comprehensive search of all journals on MEDLINE for one year failed to find more than an occasional study. Where such studies exist, often they concern decision making by nursing home personnel rather than studies of residents.

Future Directions and Conclusions

Primary care research in long-term care settings is still very much in the developmental stage. Pursuing research in this setting has some unique problems, particularly ethical; nonetheless, primary care researchers have no less reason than do subspecialists to design and implement studies in this area. A number of topics of particular importance to primary care clinicians in this field are either unexplored or inadequately explored, such as the following: (a) determinants of good or poor quality of life in institutional settings, (b) interaction of family, residents, and staff as it impacts on care, (c) approaches to the care of particular illnesses in the long-term care setting, and (d) appropriate indications for hospitalization. In particular, integrating information about quality of life and expected illness outcome can enable clinicians to make better decisions about appropriate care (Mehr, Foxman, & Colombo, 1992).

In addition to many inadequately explored topics, we do not know how much the results of existing research in nursing homes have been shaped by the preponderant use of academically affiliated teaching nursing homes and veterans' nursing homes. Only high-quality studies, performed in community settings, in the context of usual care will provide the answer. Furthermore residential care settings, which are intermediate between nursing homes and the community, are basically uninvestigated. Moving into these new settings and considering these unexplored issues is the task that lies ahead for the primary care researcher in the long-term care setting.

References

Annas, G. J., & Glantz, L. H. (1986). Rules for research in nursing homes [editorial]. *New England Journal of Medicine, 315*(18), 1157-1158.

Applegate, W. B., Blass, J. P., & Williams, T. F. (1990). Instruments for the functional assessment of older patients. *New England Journal of Medicine, 322*(17), 1207-1214.

Beecher, H. K. (1966). Ethics and clinical research. *New England Journal of Medicine, 274*, 1354-1360.

Cassel, C. K. (1985). Research in nursing homes: Ethical issues. *Journal of the American Geriatric Society, 33*(11), 795-799.

Cassel, C. K. (1987). Informed consent for research in geriatrics: History and concepts. *Journal of the American Geriatric Society, 35*(6), 542-544.

Eish, J. S., Colling, J., Ouslander, J., Hadley, B. J., & Campbell, E. (1991). Issues in implementing clinical research in nursing home settings. *Journal of the New York State Nurses Association, 122*(3), 18-22.

Hing, E. (1989). Nursing home utilization by current residents: United States, 1985. National Center for Health Statistics. *Vital and Health Statistics, 13*(102), 1-86.

Hoffman, P. B., Marron, K. R., Fillit, H., & Libow, L. S. (1983). Obtaining informed consent in the teaching nursing home. *Journal of the American Geriatric Society, 31*(9), 565-569.

Hu, T. W., Igou, J. F., Kaltreider, D. L., Yu, L., Rohner, T. J., Dennis, P. J., Craighead, E., Hadley, E. C., & Ory, M. G. (1989). A clinical trial of a behavioral therapy to reduce urinary incontinence in nursing homes. *Journal of the American Medical Association, 261*(18), 2656-2662.

Kafonek, S., Ettinger, W. H., Roca, R., Kittner, S., Taylor, N., & German, P. S. (1989). Instruments for screening for depression and dementia in a long-term care facility. *Journal of the American Geriatric Society, 37*(1), 29-34.

Kaye, J. M., Lawton, P., & Kaye, D. (1990). Attitudes of elderly people about clinical research on aging. *The Gerontologist, 30*(1), 100-106.

Keeler, E. B., Kane, R. L., & Solomon, D. H. (1981). Short- and long-term residents of nursing homes. *Medical Care, 19*(3), 363-369.

Kemper, P., & Murtaugh, C. M. (1991). Lifetime use of nursing home care. *New England Journal of Medicine, 324*(9), 595-600.

Lipsitz, L. A., Pluchino, F. C., & Wright, S. M. (1987). Biomedical research in the nursing home: Methodological issues and subject recruitment results. *Journal of the American Geriatric Society, 35*(7), 629-634.

Mehr, D. R., Foxman, B., & Colombo, P. (1992). Risk factors for mortality from lower respiratory infections in nursing home patients. *Journal of Family Practice, 34*(5), 585-591.

Melnick, V., Dubler, N. N., Weisbard, A., & Butler, R. N. (1984). Clinical research in senile dementia of the Alzheimer type: Suggested guidelines addressing the ethical and legal issues. *Journal of the American Geriatric Society, 32*, 531-536.

Morris, J. N., Hawes, C., Murphy, K., & Nonemaker, S. (1991). *Minimum data set. Resident assessment instrument training manual and resource guide.* Natick, MA: Eliot.

Warren, J. W., Sobal, J., Tenney, J. H., Hoopes, J. M., Damron, D., Levenson, S., DeForge, B. R., & Muncie, H. L., Jr. (1986). Informed consent by proxy: An issue in research with elderly patients. *New England Journal of Medicine, 30, 315*(18), 1124-1128.

Wayne, S. J., Rhyne, R. L., Thompson, R. E., & Davis, M. (1991). Sampling issues in nursing home research. *Journal of the American Geriatric Society, 39*(3), 308-311.

18 Primary Care Research in the Community

NANCY EDWARDS

Conducting relevant and methodologically sound research in the community is a crucial prerequisite for the design and implementation of effective primary care programs. In this chapter I discuss approaches that may be used to strengthen the design and enhance the feasibility of such research. Examples are drawn from a variety of community health settings where elements of primary care are provided.

Paradigms for Primary Care Research in the Community

Changes are occurring in the primary care practice setting that have important implications for research. During the last decade, we have shifted from a one-on-one emphasis where the individual or family was the client, to a community-as-client orientation, otherwise known as community-oriented primary care. Now a third paradigm is emerging: that of the community as a partner.

Each of these paradigms of service delivery has stimulated new ways of thinking about old problems, and inherent in each is a set of research questions with a particular orientation. For example, consistent with the first paradigm (individual or family as client) are questions such as: What are physician practices for the medical care of patients with diabetes mellitus (Jacques et al.,

1991)? What treatment approaches for acute low back pain are effective (Gilbert, Taylor, Hildebrand, & Evans, 1985)? What are the meanings present in the narratives of elderly hip-fracture patients (Borkan, Quirk, & Sullivan, 1991)? What are the predictors of breast self-examination among family practice patients (Norman & Tudiver, 1986)?

One of the fundamental differences between the individual-as-client versus the community-as-client orientation is the breadth of assessment in the latter. The community-as-client paradigm applies techniques of epidemiology, social sciences, and health services (Nutting & Connor, 1986; Starfield, 1991) to enhance problem definition in the community and to provide data that are more representative than those derived from clients who use the primary care system. This paradigm leads us to ask who uses our services and how do we make our services more accessible to those who do not? It thereby adds another dimension to our research questions; that is, what are the health patterns of community members, and how do we provide services that are accessible to all? Examples of studies that are consistent with this orientation include a comparison of strategies to screen for hypertension in the community (Birkett, 1991), intervention studies designed to maintain the functional capacity of seniors in the community by increasing the number of home care services available (Chambers et al., 1990), determining the accessibility of cervical screening programs (Ciatto, Cecchini, Bonardi, Venturini, & Ciacci, 1991), and prevalence studies of self-care medication practices (Segall, 1990).

Central to the community-as-partner paradigm is the concept of *community mobilization;* that is, how do we work in partnership with local individuals and organizations to facilitate action that will create an environment that supports health? The types of questions that arise with this paradigm include: What strategies effectively mobilize a community to take preventive health action, what public policies support healthful life-style choices, and how does one work in partnership with ethnic groups and organizations to increase the cultural sensitivity of primary care programs?

These three paradigms are complementary, and together they suggest an array of questions to be considered in mounting primary care community studies. An example helps illustrate this point. Using all three paradigms, we are exploring the following research questions in a community study aimed at reducing the incidence of falls among residents of seniors' apartment buildings:

1. Do home visits by a "fall-prevention" team to seniors at high risk for falls increase self-efficacy for fall prevention and reduce the incidence of falls? (Individual as Client)
2. What proportion of residents will attend a "falls clinic"? What are the characteristics of these individuals, and how do they differ from those who choose not to attend? (Community as Client)
3. Do community mobilization strategies in seniors' apartment buildings increase self- and collective efficacy for fall prevention and reduce the incidence of falls? (Community as Partner)

Although all three paradigms may be considered in the design of a research study, the last has received the least attention in the primary care literature. The remainder of this chapter focuses on primary care research that reflects this paradigm.

Strategies for Primary Care Research Using the Community-as-Partner Paradigm

The domain of questions embodied in the community-as-partner paradigm poses a number of challenges for primary care researchers. Those considered here are (a) obtaining the community perspective on a problem, (b) defining and sampling the study population, (c) measuring community participation, and (d) developing a standardized community mobilization intervention. Approaches that may be used to tackle these challenges are described, and organizational partnerships that may help support them are highlighted.

OBTAINING THE COMMUNITY PERSPECTIVE ON A PROBLEM

One should never assume that lay community members construct health-related events in the same way as health professionals. To obtain the community perspective on a health problem, it may be useful to choose a combination of qualitative and quantitative methods. Qualitative methods often allow one to obtain data that have a richness that may be lacking when quantitative methods alone are used.

For example, in preparation for our study on falls, we decided to use qualitative methods to learn how seniors themselves described the problem of falls among their age group. We carried out a series of ethnographic interviews and focus groups with noninstitutionalized seniors who resided in both rural and urban communities. During these interviews we asked questions concerning their personal experience with falls, what they thought increased their chances of falling, and what they thought could be done to prevent falls.

These interviews revealed some important perceptions. First, although our respondents correctly identified many of the risk factors cited in the research literature, their reports frequently reflected a sense of fatalism toward this problem, as illustrated in the following descriptions: "It just happened," "I was down before I knew what hit me," or "It was just carelessness." Second, their descriptions of major risk factors differed from those found in the literature. Medication misuse and polypharmacy, for example, were rarely identified as important risk factors, while wearing inappropriate footwear was frequently cited as a hazard. Third, their descriptions of falls revealed some reticence to admit to having fallen. For example, one respondent stated: "I did fall once, but I was just down and right back up again." Even when they were given a definition of a fall, many persisted in using their own notion of what constituted one. One woman stated that she had not fallen for many years; then she commented that "everyone slips on the ice." When asked whether she had slipped on the ice, she said that she had and had landed on her bottom. However, throughout the interview she continued to maintain that her slip on the ice was not a fall. Later in the interview, she described her fear of being institutionalized.

Use of the qualitative methods provided other insights. For example, focus groups were organized in seniors' apartment buildings. Because of consistently poor turnouts for other group events in these buildings, we had some concerns that residents would be reticent to attend these sessions; however, virtually all who were invited did attend, and in many cases they brought others along. The focus group discussions were very animated, and participants expressed enthusiasm for having been asked to share their views on the problem rather than just being told what to do by a health professional. It became clear that focus groups not only were useful as a means of data collection but also could be used as an approach with the senior population to help build community awareness around the problem of falls.

During these focus group sessions, seniors were asked to share their views on and experiences with the use of a buddy system in apartment buildings. Our research team thought the use of such a system would be an appropriate strategy in apartment buildings, so that an individual who had suffered a serious fall would be found quickly. Although some residents thought this was a good idea, the response was by no means consistent. A number of residents considered this to be butting into other people's business and wanted no part of it. This illustrates the discrepancy that may exist between what health providers and clients view as appropriate strategies to support healthful living in the community.

This qualitative data on seniors' perceptions of falls laid the groundwork for a variety of research activities, including developing an instrument to measure attitudes toward fall prevention, delineating a series of questions to use as probes to obtain retrospective data on falls, selecting a theoretical basis for a fall-prevention program, and identifying community mobilization strategies for fall prevention.

The primary care setting can afford many opportunities to talk with clients about their perceptions of health-related problems, and it is important that we take the time to find ways to understand the clients who are the targets of our services. These initiatives may be critical to the development of effective interventions and the measurement of appropriate outcomes in a study.

DEFINING AND SAMPLING
THE STUDY POPULATION

Defining the study population within a community-as-partner paradigm requires that we think beyond the "clinic" population. With respect to any health problem, it is important that we consider individuals both directly and indirectly affected by the problem as potential target groups. For example, if a study population

has been defined rather crudely as the "frail elderly," many
questions need to be asked concerning the frail elderly who do
not regularly come into contact with primary care services, and
the relationships between these people and other community
members. A few examples: How do community members recognize frailty? Where do the frail elderly reside, and how quickly
do they become connected with primary care service providers
after a crisis? Other than health professionals, who provides support for them? Working with community residents and with other
service providers to explore their perceptions of a health problem
will help ensure that an operational definition of the study population is well grounded in the community reality of the problem.

Having defined a study population, one then must select a suitable sampling technique. For those studies that require a random
sample of the population, it will be necessary to identify an accessible and accurate sampling frame and an affordable sampling
strategy. Rarely are up-to-date lists of primary care clinic atten-
dees the first choice for selecting a representative sample of
community residents. The reason for this lies in the potential bias
introduced by excluding those who choose not to use such services.
Examples of alternative sampling frames available to researchers
are tax assessment or electoral rolls, telephone directories, and
comprehensive lists compiled by community organizations. It is
important to consider what population subgroups may be underrepresented or excluded in each potential sampling frame. In
some situations it will be necessary to compile a sampling frame
by conducting a census of the population of interest.

When it is necessary to sample rare population units such as
minority ethnic groups, the cost of sampling from a list of all community members increases enormously, and so many of those
initially sampled will have to be discarded from the study because they do not meet the eligibility criteria. Techniques have been
developed to increase sampling efficiency for rare population
units (Blair & Czaja, 1982; Inglis, Groves, & Heeringa, 1987).

Sampling procedures for qualitative studies do not require
such rigorous attention to representativeness. The objectives of
the study and the research design will guide the choice of an
appropriate sampling strategy.

MEASURING COMMUNITY PARTICIPATION

Many of the research questions that emerge from a community-as-partner paradigm focus on a process of community mobilization. Selecting outcome measures that allow us to quantify the outcomes of this process or the process itself is challenging. Some measures are available to examine the outcomes of community participation—for example, dimensions of a supportive environment such as the presence of public policies (Pederson, Bull, Ashley, & Lefcoe, 1986), measures of social support (Bernard et al., 1990), neighborhood cohesion (Buckner, 1988), and collective efficacy (Edwards, Murphy, Birkett, Nair, & Corber, 1991). However, instruments to measure the process of community mobilization are much less common.

Rifkin, Muller, and Bichmann (1988) described the use of a pentagram model to assess community participation. Five factors that influence the participation process are included: needs assessment, leadership, organization, resource mobilization, and management. Process indicators can be identified for each of the factors, and a continuum is developed for each of these indicators with the following anchor points: wide community participation with professionals acting as resources, and narrow participation where professionals make all decisions with no community participation. The pentagram then can be used to monitor various aspects of community participation in a primary care program (Bjaras, Haglund, & Rifkin, 1991).

The qualitative literature is replete with data collection methods that lend themselves to describing the process of community mobilization and participation. These methods may be helpful used either alone or in conjunction with quantitative techniques. We have found the use of field notes to be a particularly helpful documentation strategy. Clinicians are shown how to keep field notes and are asked to write them during both pilot testing of study instruments and interventions and during the implementation phase of studies designed to test the effectiveness of interventions. As such note taking is time-consuming, it is critical that clear objectives for field notes be delineated and time frames for a review of them be established.

DESCRIBING THE INTERVENTION AND
DETERMINING STANDARDIZATION

A cornerstone of good research design for intervention studies is the need to standardize study interventions. Without this step, both the internal and external validity of a study are threatened. However, designing a community mobilization intervention that can be tested in a research study is difficult. These interventions lack many of the easily described features of more traditional interventions such as drug trials or packaged health education sessions, which are uniformly applied to all clients. The nature of community mobilization interventions requires that the intervention be adjusted to fit the characteristics of particular clients or subgroups in the population.

Prior to standardizing an intervention, it may be useful to ascertain what approaches clinicians currently use in particular situations. For example, we have employed long interviews with clinicians to determine what strategies they use to prevent falls among seniors. To elicit responses, clinicians were presented with several scenarios where certain patient characteristics were varied (e.g., cognitive impairment, age, frailty) and were asked to describe how they would try to elicit specific behavior changes. This type of data helps shed light on the amount of variability already present in the way clinicians tackle particular community health problems. This information is vital in determining what aspects of an intervention need to be standardized and in planning training sessions for clinicians to prepare them to implement a standardized intervention.

An explicit description of the conceptual framework underlying the study intervention is an essential prerequisite to the standardization process. The conceptual framework sets clear parameters for the major components of an intervention. It also serves to guide the amount of latitude that clinicians can use in adjusting the intervention to fit a particular group. An important aspect of training clinicians to carry out the intervention involves ensuring that they are readily able to apply the key elements of the conceptual framework in a variety of situations. It is the strategies aimed at changing individual, community, and organizational behaviors that are often the critical pieces of a commu-

nity mobilization intervention. These strategies will arise out of
the conceptual framework and must be described clearly.

ORGANIZATIONAL PARTNERSHIPS
THAT SUPPORT RESEARCH
IN THE PRACTICE SETTING

Fundamental to successful research in the community are strong
organizational partnerships. A buying-in process is required to
get both community members and practitioners supportive of
research projects. This approach has a number of potential pitfalls. As an example, our study of falls among seniors required
that we keep nurses closely informed of the results of the pilot
studies and funding status of this project because they will be
responsible for implementing the intervention. Interestingly fall
prevention was not an intervention that had featured strongly in
the nurses' practice prior to the development of this research
initiative. However, the attention it attracted as we shared our
pilot work with them peaked their interest in the problem, and
the resultant difficulty has been trying to minimize the risk of
their co-intervention.

Our approach to this potential problem has involved establishing mechanisms to help service providers (both frontline workers
and management) recognize when and how service delivery
decisions can affect research. Nurses have been encouraged to
contact a member of the research team whenever they need to
check whether an activity they propose in the community could
potentially act as a co-intervention. A survey has been conducted
of nurses to determine what interventions are currently in place
regarding fall prevention, thus serving as a baseline and also as
a reminder to nurses about the co-intervention issue.

Partnerships with other community agencies involved in various aspects of service delivery to seniors have allowed us to negotiate which seniors' apartment buildings will be "kept clean" for
our study and which will be used for other surveys and projects.
Open dialogue has been achieved by including key members of
community agencies on a research advisory committee and by
making presentations to relevant organizations. A critical component of these relationships has been helping our partners

differentiate between what is an optimal *clinical* or program-based decision and what is a desirable *research* decision.

We have found it useful to remember that although the expertise of the clinician is essential, it is important that one consider alternatives that may be outside or contrary to this professional's experience. For example, in deciding to conduct a cross-sectional survey of residents in seniors' buildings, we were strongly advised by nurses not to conduct the survey during the month of June, as in their experience the response would be very low. Nurses had found that attendance at clinics and group sessions markedly declined as summer approached. In this particular situation, we did not have a choice, as personnel availability for the research project required that we conduct the survey in June. Our results (Edwards, Hughes, LeBlond, Caloren, & MacNamara, 1990) were very different from those projected by the nurses: Out of a random sample of 525 seniors in 25 different apartment buildings, we attained a contact rate of 94% and a response rate of 88.9%. This example illustrates that it is useful to consider the guidance provided by service providers but that clinicians may misjudge a response to a research project because it is outside their realm of experience.

Summary

In conclusion, the community-as-partner paradigm holds both promise and challenges for those interested in conducting research in the practice setting. Identifying and using opportunities for conducting such research can help both practitioners and community members expand their thinking about ways to tackle health-related problems.

References

Bernard, H. R., Johnsen, E. C., Killworth, P. D., McCarty, C., Shelley, G. A., & Robinson, S. (1990). Comparing four different methods for measuring personal social networks. *Social Networks, 12*, 179-215.

Birkett, N. J. (1991, November). *Using community blood pressure screening clinics to assess hypertension control and prevalence.* Paper presented at the Annual Meeting of the American Public Health Association, Atlanta, GA.

Bjaras, G., Haglund, B. J. A., & Rifkin, S. B. (1991). A new approach to community participation assessment. *Health Promotion International, 6*(3), 199-206.

Blair, J., & Czaja, R. (1982). Locating a special population using random digit dialing. *Public Opinion Quarterly, 46,* 585-590.

Borkan, J. M., Quirk, M., & Sullivan, M. (1991). Finding meaning after the fall: Injury narratives from elderly hip fracture patients. *Social Science and Medicine, 33*(8), 947-957.

Buckner, J. C. (1988). Neighborhood Cohesion Instrument. *Journal of Community Psychology, 16*(6), 771-791.

Chambers, L. W., Tugwell, P., Goldsmith, C. H., Caulfield, P., Haight, M., Pickard, L., & Gibbon, M. (1990). The impact of home care on recently discharged elderly hospital patients in an Ontario community. *Canadian Journal of Aging, 4,* 327-347.

Ciatto, S., Cecchini, S., Bonardi, R., Venturini, A., & Ciacci, R. (1991). Attendance to a screening program for cervical cancer in the city of Florence. *Tumori, 77*(3), 252-256.

Edwards, N., Hughes, L., LeBlond, D., Caloren, H., & MacNamara, M. (1990, June). *A community assessment of the needs of seniors' apartment building residents in Ottawa—Opportunities for innovative practice.* Paper presented at the Annual Meeting of the Canadian Association of University Schools of Nursing National Nursing Research Conference, Victoria, B.C.

Edwards, N., Murphy, M., Birkett, N., Nair, R., & Corber, S. (1991). *A randomized controlled trial of the effectiveness of two strategies to reduce the incidence of falls among seniors.* Unpublished research grant. Ontario Ministry of Health.

Gilbert, J. R., Taylor, D. W., Hildebrand, A., & Evans, C. (1985). Clinical trial of common treatments for low back pain in family practice. *British Medical Journal of Clinical Research, 291*(6498), 771-774.

Inglis, K. M., Groves, R. M., & Heeringa, S. G. (1987). Telephone sample designs for the U.S. black household population. *Survey Methodology, 13*(1), 1-14.

Jacques, C. H., Jones, R. L., Houts, P., Bauer, L. C., Dwyer, K. M., Lynch, J. C., & Casale, T. S. (1991). Reported practice behaviors for medical care of patients with diabetes mellitus by primary-care physicians in Pennsylvania. *Diabetes Care, 14*(8), 712-717.

Norman, R. M., & Tudiver, F. (1986). Predictors of breast self-examination among family practice patients. *Journal of Family Practice, 22*(2), 149-153.

Nutting, P., & Connor, E. (1986). Community-oriented primary care: An integrated model for practice, research, and education. *American Journal of Preventive Medicine, 2,* 140-147.

Pederson, L. L., Bull, S. B., Ashley, M. J., & Lefcoe, N. M. (1986). A population survey on legislative measures to restrict smoking in Ontario. *American Journal of Preventive Medicine, 6,* 307-315.

Rifkin, S. B., Muller, F., & Bichmann, W. (1988). Primary health care: On measuring participation. *Social Science and Medicine, 26,* 931-940.

Segall, A. (1990). A community survey of self-medication activities. *Medical Care,*
    28(4), 301-310.
Starfield, B. (1991). Innovative ways to study primary care using traditional
    methods. In P. G. Norton, M. Stewart, F. Tudiver, M. J. Bass, & E. V. Dunn (Eds.),
    Primary care research: Traditional and innovative approaches (pp. 26-39). Newbury
    Park, CA: Sage.

Appendix
Checklist for Conducting Research in the Practice Setting

MARTIN J. BASS
VANESSA J. ORR

Introduction

Ravetz (1971) has defined a mature discipline as one in which the research methods are established and the pitfalls have been identified. Primary care research is still very much a growing discipline. The research methods are those of epidemiology, psychology, sociology, and anthropology, encompassing both quantitative and qualitative approaches. Many of the pitfalls have been identified.

The five volumes in the series *Research Methods for Primary Care* have identified the methods that work and some of the pitfalls to be avoided. The following is a guide to both methods and pitfalls for the interested researcher. The checklist consists of key questions that draw the researcher's attention to potential pitfalls.

Throughout the checklist are guides to further information to assist in addressing that issue. These are based primarily on the five volumes in this series, with some additional references. Other useful sources of information are standard research texts in the fields of family practice, epidemiology, statistics, and sociology.

Checklist for Conducting Research
in the Practice Setting

A. GETTING STARTED

1. Research question (see Vol. 1, Ch. 2)
   a. What is the question?
   b. Is it of interest to you?
   c. Is it answerable?
   d. Would the answer to your question enhance care?
   e. Can you do it in your setting, or do you need other practices?
   f. Can you do it with your resources?
2. Literature review
   a. Have you conducted a computer literature search?
   b. If you require help, have you contacted a librarian at a university, hospital, or family practice association?
   c. Have you examined the literature for:
      other studies answering a question similar to yours?
      important confounding factors?
      useful measures specific for your topic?
      successful methodologies?
      problems others have encountered?
   d. Have you spoken to knowledgeable colleagues?
3. Refine and focus research question (see Vol. 1, Chs. 2 & 6). Are you:
   a. repeating a published study in your setting?
   b. adding a new dimension to an already published study?
   c. exploring or testing a new hypothesis?
   d. doing a pilot or feasibility study?
4. Consultants/collaborations
   a. Could your staff/patients/allied health professionals contribute to the research question and method? (see Vol. 4, Ch. 9)
   b. Do you need the help of research consultants (statistician, epidemiologist, social scientist, family practice researcher)? (see Vol. 5, Ch. 12)
   c. If multiple researchers, are tasks and responsibilities clear? (see Vol. 5, Ch. 13)

B. STUDY DESIGN

1. Method
   a. Have you chosen an appropriate design? (see Vol. 1, Ch. 6)
      For description—surveys, audits, case studies (see Vol. 1, Chs. 4, 7, & 8; Vol. 2, Ch. 14)
      For exploring etiology—case control, cohort studies (see Vol. 1, Ch. 5)
      For evaluation—audits, cohort studies, trials (see Vol. 4, Chs. 1, 3, 6, & 10)
      For new insights—qualitative studies, detailed review of charts (see Vol. 4, Chs. 8 & 10)
   b. If a test of a new therapy, is there a comparison group and random allocation? (see Vol. 4, Chs. 1 & 3)
   c. If you are searching for etiological factors, is there a comparison group?
   d. Is the research designed to fit well with clinical care? (see Vol. 5, Ch. 4)
2. Measures
   a. Are you using a previously existing measure? If yes, are its psychometric properties known and appropriate? (equally applicable to the measurement of blood pressure or depression) (see Vol. 2, Chs. 5, 6, & Appendix)
   b. Are you developing your own measure? (see Vol. 2, Chs. 6 & 8)
   c. Are you cutting and pasting from more than one existing measure? (see Vol. 2, Ch. 9)
   d. Have you considered your outcomes and how to measure them? (see Vol. 2, Ch. 2)
3. Sample
   a. Have you done a sample size calculation (see Hulley & Cummings, 1988):
      i. looking for a clinically significant difference between two groups?
      ii. looking for proportion within a specified confidence interval?
   b. Is the sample representative?

    c. In the time allotted for the study, can one practice provide enough subjects, or are multiple practices necessary? (see Vol. 2, Ch. 7)

4. Ensuring data quality (see Vol. 1, Ch. 6)
    a. Are definitions clear?
    b. Will you have to train recorders, or can you and your staff collect the data?
    c. If chart audit, have you designed and tested an abstract form?
    d. Will you collect data in a consistent manner?
    e. Will you monitor data collection regularly?
    f. Are objective measures used wherever possible?
    g. Are the recorders blinded to patient assignment or study hypothesis?
    h. Do you have checks built into your measures to evaluate data quality?

5. Ethical considerations (see Vol. 5, Ch. 3)
    a. Do you need to submit your study to an ethical review panel, and have you allowed time for their review process?
    b. Have you made provision for obtaining informed consent based on:
      i. explanation of benefits and risks?
      ii. voluntary participation?
      iii. usual care unaffected if person chooses not to participate?
      iv. permission to withdraw at any time?
      v. assurance of confidentiality?
    c. Is a signed consent form needed?

6. Piloting
    a. Have you piloted:
      i. your study method?
      ii. your data collection instruments?
      iii. recruitment strategies, including explanations and consent forms?

7. Have you modified your study design based on the pilot?

8. Have you projected a realistic schedule or time line for the study, anticipating problems with recruitment and data analysis and overlapping of tasks?

C. RECRUITING SUBJECTS

1. Have clear and realistic inclusion and exclusion criteria been stated?
2. If a random sample is required, have you developed a comprehensive list of subjects from which the sample can be drawn?
3. Have you identified who will do the recruiting? (see Vol. 5, Chs. 4 & 5)

D. PRACTICE ORGANIZATION

1. Have you involved the practice staff by (see Vol. 4, Ch. 9):
   a. informing them of the study design and purpose?
   b. explaining the importance of their role?
   c. listening to their ideas?
   d. modifying their usual tasks or reimbursing them for extra time?
2. Is the research consistent with clinical care? (see Vol. 5, Chs. 4 & 5)
   a. Has the research protocol been streamlined to minimize its impact?
   b. Do you need additional staff to collect data?
3. Have your patients been appropriately involved?

E. DATA MANAGEMENT AND ANALYSIS
   FOR QUANTITATIVE DATA

1. Data management issues:
   a. Do you have access to either simple data management programs or more sophisticated statistical programs? (see Vol. 2, Ch. 18)
   b. Have data been entered in a manner that protects confidentiality (using identification numbers instead of names)?
   c. Have you ensured that your data entry is accurate by:
      i. using the "checking" system provided in your computer package (e.g., setting legal values/appropriate ranges for variables)?

      ii. visual inspection of a data listing and preliminary
         frequency distributions for each variable looking
         for clearly incorrect data?
      iii. exploratory graphics?

2. Preliminary issues for analysis
   a. Do you require ongoing consultation with a biostatis-
      tician, epidemiologist, or family physician researcher?
   b. Have you started your data analysis by studying the
      frequency distributions of the key variables?

3. Hypothesis testing
   a. If there are two or more groups, have you compared
      baseline characteristics to identify important differ-
      ences that may influence the interpretation of your
      results?
   b. Have you selected the appropriate statistics to test
      your hypotheses? (see Hulley & Cummings, 1988)
   c. Have you considered possible confounding variables?
   d. Have you considered statistical versus clinical sig-
      nificance? (see Vol. 4, Ch. 6)
   e. If no difference was found, could it be due to an
      insufficient sample size (low power)? (see Vol. 2, Ch. 6)

F. HANDLING AND ANALYZING
   QUALITATIVE DATA

1. Have you selected the appropriate analysis strategy?
   (see Vol. 3, Chs. 1, 5-10)
2. Have you built in adequate time and resources for ongoing transcription and data manipulation?
3. Have you arranged lengthy blocks of quiet, uninter-
   rupted time for doing the analysis?
4. Have you planned for and arranged validation activities? (see Vol. 1, Ch. 10)

G. FUNDING

1. Does the project require funding, or is it small enough
   to be done with existing resources?

2. Have you developed a comprehensive budget including as necessary:
   a. assistants (secretarial support, research personnel)?
   b. consultants?
   c. special equipment or tests?
   d. supplies (photocopying, printing, software, stamps, phone, miscellaneous)?
   e. office space, furniture?
   f. travel to collect data?
   g. travel to present results?
   h. data analysis?
   i. miscellaneous—inflation, reprints, reimbursement of subject expenses, honoraria to office staff collecting data?
3. Have you contacted any of the following for funding information:
   a. peers?
   b. nearby university department or university research office?
   c. professional organization?
   d. special interest agencies (e.g., heart, asthma, mental health)?
   e. state or national funding?
   f. foundations?
   g. pharmaceutical companies? (see Vol. 5, Ch. 11)

H. REPORTING

1. Have you shared your interpretation of the results with co-researchers, staff, and subjects? (see Vol. 5, Ch. 2)
2. If multiple authors, have you agreed on writing tasks and credits?
3. Are you disseminating your results widely:
   a. via oral presentation
   b. writing and submitting a journal article (see Huth, 1990)
   c. discussing your results with the media

References

Hulley, S. B., & Cummings, S. R. (1988). *Designing clinical research.* Baltimore: Williams & Wilkins.

Huth, J. (1990). *How to write and publish papers in the medical sciences* (2nd ed.). Baltimore: Williams & Wilkins.

Ravetz, J. R. (1971). *Scientific knowledge and its social problems.* New York: Oxford University Press.

Volumes in the series *Research Methods for Primary Care:*

Norton, P. G., Stewart, M., Tudiver, F., Bass, M. J., & Dunn, E. V. (Eds.). (1991). *Research methods for primary care: Vol. 1. Primary care research: Traditional and innovative approaches.* Newbury Park, CA: Sage.

Stewart, M., Tudiver, F., Bass, M. J., Dunn, E. V., & Norton, P. G. (Eds.). (1992). *Research methods for primary care: Vol. 2. Tools for primary care research.* Newbury Park, CA: Sage.

Crabtree, B. F., & Miller, W. L. (Eds.). (1992). *Research methods for primary care: Vol. 3. Doing qualitative research.* Newbury Park, CA: Sage.

Tudiver, F., Bass, M. J., Dunn, E. V., Norton, P. G., & Stewart, M. (Eds.). (1992). *Research methods for primary care: Vol. 4. Assessing interventions: Traditional and innovative methods.* Newbury Park, CA: Sage.

Bass, M. J., Dunn, E. V., Norton, P. G., Stewart, M., & Tudiver, F. (Eds.). (1993). *Research methods for primary care: Vol. 5. Conducting research in the practice setting.* Newbury Park, CA: Sage.

Index

About the Authors

Giora Almagor (MD, FRCGP) was a Consultant in Primary Health Care at the World Health Organization Regional Office for Europe and is the current Chair of the Council of WONCA—World Organization of Family Doctors—and convener of a working party to promote general practice/family medicine in China. He is a trainer at the Rommema Teaching Clinic in Israel and Director of the Northern Branch of the National Institute for Training in Family Medicine and Primary Care.

Martin J. Bass (MD, MSc, CCFP) is Professor of Family Medicine and Epidemiology at The University of Western Ontario in London, Canada. He is Director of the Centre for Studies in Family Medicine. Since joining the Department of Family Medicine in 1973, He has concentrated on improving the research base of family practice and the development of appropriate research methods. He directed the first Masters program for family medicine academics. He has been a visiting professor at Perth, Utrecht, Harvard, and Israel. His research includes treatment of hypertension in family practice, technology applications in family practice, implementing prevention in practice, and quality of care. He is the current holder of the McWhinney Chair for Research in Family Medicine.

Marie-Dominique Beaulieu (MD, MSc, CCFP) is a Professor in the Department of Family Practice of the University of Montreal and has been a member of the Canadian Task Force on the Periodic

Health Examination since 1984. After completing her family medicine residency at Laval University, in Quebec, in 1978, she studied at the Kellogg Centre for Advanced Studies in Primary Care, affiliated to McGill University, in Montreal. She completed her master's degree in epidemiology in 1982. Her research interests are the implementation of preventive programs in the practice setting and evaluation of the impact of continuity of care and medical information systems.

Jeffrey M. Borkan (MD, PhD) is Assistant Professor of Family and Community Medicine at the University of Massachusetts Medical Center; Director of Research in Family Medicine at Ben-Gurion University in Israel; and a Lecturer in Behavioral Science and the Coordinator of the Israeli Family Practice Research Network. He is a medical anthropologist and practicing rural family physician who, for the last decade, has straddled two fields and two continents. His academic training has taken him from the University of Michigan and Hebrew University to Case Western Reserve, the University of Washington, and Harvard. His areas of interest include qualitative research, narrative analysis, health beliefs, hip fractures, and low back pain.

Judith Belle Brown (PhD) is an Assistant Professor in the Department of Family Medicine at The University of Western Ontario and the Department of Social Work at King's College. She conducts research in the areas of doctor-patient communication, physician well-being, family physician-specialist communication, and wife abuse. She is known nationally for her workshops on the patient-centered method of practice and small group teaching.

Nancy Edwards (BScN, MSc) is an Assistant Professor of Nursing and a Researcher in the Community Health Research Unit, a joint project of the University of Ottawa and the Ottawa-Carleton Health Department. Her community health experience has been in diverse settings, including Newfoundland, Pakistan, Sierra Leone, and Ontario. Her research interests include fall prevention among seniors, multicultural health, decision making for self-care, and the application of research findings in community health nursing practice.

Eugene Farley (MD, MPH) is Professor and Chair of the Department of Family Medicine and Practice, University of Wisconsin. After obtaining his MPH from Johns Hopkins, he started and headed the Family Medicine Program at the University of Rochester and Highland Hospital (1967-1978) and was Chair of Family Medicine at the University of Colorado (1978-1982). His interests include developing "practices as laboratories"; developing systems that facilitate patient care, research, education, and practice management; clarifying the importance of the general practice function and family practice function in the clinical care of individuals and families by family physicians; educating medical students and physicians in the clinical specialty of Family Practice; and improving the accessibility and availability of health/medical care for everyone.

William L. Freeman (MD, MPH) is Director of the Indian Health Service Research Program in Tucson and Director of Research and Institutional Review Board of the Indian Health Service in Tucson. He was an English major (Amherst College), Peace Corps volunteer (Columbia University), independent-duty medic in Vietnam (U.S. Army's Special Forces "Green Berets"), and Deputy Director of Medex (for ex-independent-duty medics to become physician assistants). At the University of Washington in Seattle he received his MD and MPH and completed Family Medicine residency. He was a family physician at Lummi Indian Reservation, Bellingham, Washington, for 13 years. His interests include practice-based research and research ethics.

Lillian Gelberg (MD, MSPH) is Assistant Professor in the Division of Family Medicine, University of California at Los Angeles. She received her BA in Psychobiology from UCLA in 1977 and her MD from Harvard Medical School in 1981. She obtained her family medicine training in the Social Medicine Residency Program of Montefiore Hospital in the Bronx, New York, in 1984. She had a 2-year fellowship at the UCLA Robert Wood Johnson Clinical Scholars Program, during which she obtained a MSPH in Health Services Research in 1986. Her research interests include predictors of health status, use of health services, and compliance with medical care among the homeless and other impoverished populations.

Toula M. Gerace (RN, BScN) is a Clinical Lecturer in the Department of Family Medicine, The University of Western Ontario. She is a family practice nurse. Her clinical and research interests are in health promotion, disease prevention, and a special interest in the area of collaboration. She has presented workshops and research findings at local and national meetings and has been published in such journals as *Family Medicine,* the *Journal of Medical Education,* and the *Canadian Family Physician.* She currently is completing her thesis toward an MSc in Epidemiology at The University of Western Ontario.

Brian Hennen (MD, MA, CCFP, FCFP, FRCGP) is Chair of the Department of Family Medicine at The University of Western Ontario. He is a certificant and fellow of the College of Family Physicians of Canada, of which he is a past president. He has studied the teaching of ethics to medical students and co-teaches Ethical Issues in Family Medicine, a course for family medicine and philosophy graduate students.

Carol P. Herbert (MD, CCFP, FCFP) is Royal Canadian Legion Professor and Head of the Department of Family Practice at the University of British Columbia. She is a certificant and fellow of the College of Family Physicians of Canada. She has been the YWCA Woman of Distinction in Health and Social Sciences, a member of the National Research Committee, Chair of the B.C. Chapter Research Committee, Chair of the NRC, and President of the Board of NAPCRG. Her research questions have been spawned by her practice experience. Her current research is focused on assault and sexual abuse, and the development of community-based research.

John Hickner (MD) is Associate Professor of Family Medicine at the Michigan State University College of Human Medicine. After completing his Family Practice Residency in Charleston, South Carolina, he was recruited to the rural north woods of Michigan to teach for the innovative Upper Peninsula Medical Education Program. He was Assistant Director for Undergraduate Education for 9 years. He has been involved extensively in practice-based and network research during the past 8 years. He is co-founder of the Michigan Research Network (MIRNET), board member of the Ambulatory Sentinel Practice Network (ASPN), and Director of the Upper Peninsula Research Network (UPRNet). His research interests have focused on smoking cessation in pregnancy, fluoride supplementation for caries prevention, and recruitment and retention of family physicians in rural areas.

John R. Hilditch (MD, MPH, CCFP) is Associate Professor in the Primary Care Research Unit, Department of Family and Community Medicine, Sunnybrook Health Science Centre, University of Toronto; and Associate Professor in the Department of Family and Community Medicine, University of Toronto, attached to the Sunnybrook Health Science Centre and working at the Primary Care Research Unit. He has conducted research in the areas of hypertension, menopause, and quality of life. In his work with the pharmaceutical industry, he has coordinated a data collection center for four multicenter trials, has been the principal investigator for two single-center trials, and has been consultant for one other.

William E. Hogg (HonBSc, MSc, MD, CM, FCFP) is Assistant Professor, Department of Family Medicine, University of Ottawa. He received his medical undergraduate education at McGill University, completed his residency training in Family Medicine at The University of Western Ontario, and practiced in a small community for 14 years. His research interests are in small hospital obstetrics and computers and preventive medicine.

Jacques Lemelin (MD) is Assistant Professor in the Department of Family Medicine at the University of Ottawa and Clinical Researcher at the Clinical Epidemiology Unit at the University of Ottawa. He is also Chair of the Computer User Group of the University of Ottawa and Research Coordinator at the Melrose Family Practice Unit. He joined the Department of Family Medicine, University of Ottawa, in 1990, after 13 years of practice in a small rural community. His research interests are depression, medical informatics, and continuity of care.

Joseph H. Levenstein (MD) is Professor and Head of the Department of Family and Community Medicine, University of Illinois College of Medicine at Rockford. He was formerly Head of the Unit of General Practice at the University of Cape Town. Author of 60 papers, receiver of several awards, and speaker and visiting professor throughout the world, he has held several committee positions on WONCA. His principal interests include research and medical education.

Ann C. Macaulay (MD, CCFP) is Associate Professor in the Department of Family Medicine, McGill University, and an advisor to National Health and Welfare Canada for issues regarding diabetes in Canada's aboriginal population. She graduated in 1966 from St. Andrew's University, Scotland; was hired by the Native Mohawk Community of Kahnawake, Quebec, as the founding physician of the first Native-controlled health care center in Canada; and remained there as medical director until 1988. There she conducted community-based research in both diabetes and breast-feeding and developed expertise in returning these results to the community. She continues with research and some direct patient care in Kahnawake.

Carol McWilliam (EdD) is Assistant Professor in the Departments of Family Medicine and Nursing, The University of Western Ontario. She conducts research on health promotion and health services delivery and is developing new applications of qualitative methods in research on innovative care strategies, program evaluation, and interdisciplinary dynamics related to both institutional and community-based care.

David R. Mehr (MD, MS) is Assistant Professor in the Department of Family and Community Medicine, University of Missouri-Columbia. He completed undergraduate and medical education in California, a Family Practice residency at the University of Missouri-Columbia, and practiced in Columbia for 9 years. He was certified in Geriatric Medicine in 1988. After completing a fellowship in Geriatric Medicine and an MS in Clinical Research Design and Statistical Analysis at the University of Michigan, he joined their Family Practice Department before assuming his present position. Research interests include nursing home infections, predictors of outcome of nursing home care, and preventive services in the elderly.

Brian Morris (MD, CCFP, FCFP) is Assistant Professor in the Department of Family and Community Medicine, University of Toronto. He was educated at the University of Toronto, did his Family Practice residency at St. Michael's Hospital, and is now a Community Research Consultant there. His research interests include microresearch methodologies, prevention, and community advocacy.

Paul A. Nutting (MD, MSPH) is Deputy Director of the Center for General Health Services Research and the Director of the Division of Primary Care within the Center. He was educated at Cornell University and received his MD degree from the University of Kansas and an MS in Epidemiology and Biometry from the University of Colorado. He has residency training in Pediatrics at the Children's Hospital of Pittsburgh, Preventive Medicine at the University of Arizona, and Family Medicine at the Mercy Medical Center in Denver. His research interests lie in assessing quality of care, decision analysis, automated health records, clinical preventive services, and community-oriented primary care.

Vanessa J. Orr (MA) is a Lecturer in the Department of Family Medicine, and the Research Associate and Facilitator for The Centre for Studies in Family Medicine at The University of Western Ontario. She has expertise in questionnaire design, research methodology, and analysis and currently is conducting research in the area of patient information needs.

John F. Sangster (MD, MClSc, CCFP, FCFP) is a Professor in the Department of Family Medicine, Medical Director of the Byron Family Medical Centre (Teaching Practice), and Chair of the Graduate Studies Program in Family Medicine at The University of Western Ontario. He received his MD from The University of Western Ontario, completed residency training in family medicine at St. Joseph's Hospital, and for 8 years was in private practice. His major research interest focuses on collaborative practice-based research in the areas of prevention and health promotion.

Nigel C. H. Stott (BSc, MB, FRCP, FRCGP) is Professor and Head, Department of General Practice, University of Wales, U.K. He was appointed to the Welsh Chair in 1986. His research has included a decade investigating, with anthropologist R. Pill, the health choices and behavior of working class Welsh families.